FIRST STEPS IN RESEARCH:
A Pocketbook for Healthcare Students

For Elsevier:

Commissioning Editor: Heidi Harrison
Associate Editor: Siobhan Campbell
Development Editor: Veronika Krcilova
Production Manager: Joannah Duncan
Design: Sarah Russell

FIRST STEPS IN RESEARCH:
A Pocketbook for Healthcare Students

By
Stuart Porter
BSc (Hons), Grad Dip Phys, MCSP, SRP, Cert MHS

Foreword
By
Rosie Hunt
BA (Hons), student physiotherapist

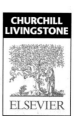

CHURCHILL
LIVINGSTONE

ELSEVIER

EDINBURGH LONDON NEW YORK OXFORD
PHILADELPHIA ST LOUIS SYDNEY TORONTO 2008

CHURCHILL
LIVINGSTONE
ELSEVIER

An imprint of Elsevier Limited

First published 2008

© 2008, Elsevier Ltd

ISBN   978-0-443-10398-8

British Library Cataloguing in Publication Data
A catalogue record for this book is available from the British Library.

Library of Congress Cataloging in Publication Data
A catalog record for this book is available from the Library of
Congress.

Note
Neither the Publisher nor the Authors assume any responsibility for
any loss or injury and/or damage to persons or property arising out
of or related to any use of the material contained in this book. It is
the responsibility of the treating practitioner, relying on independent
expertise and knowledge of the patient, to determine the best
treatment and method of application for the patient.

Printed in China

CONTENTS

For my nieces Alyssa, Lucy and Natasha and my parents Brian and Winifred who have tirelessly given their all and encouraged me without fail; my fantastic daughters, all of whom I have loved since the first day I saw them, who taught me about the fairies at the bottom of the garden and helped me to see Santa Claus. I am very proud to be called Dad; and for my wife Sue for juggling it all! Also for Reggie.

Stuart Porter graduated as a Chartered Physiotherapist from Manchester Royal Infirmary in 1987 and worked in Lancashire in Orthopaedics and Rheumatology. He began lecturing in 1997 at the University of Salford and started his PhD in 2000, looking at the determinants of exercise behaviour in people with ankylosing spondylitis. He now lives in Lancashire with his wife and three daughters.

Also by this author:

The Anatomy Workbook
ISBN 0750654554
Butterworth Heinemann

Tidy's Physiotherapy 13th edn.
ISBN: 0750632119
Butterworth Heinemann

Dictionary of Physiotherapy
ISBN 0750688335
Butterworth Heinemann

I first encountered Stuart Porter sitting on a desk at the front of our class, swinging his legs and talking about the anatomy of the lower limb. This was my first ever physiotherapy lecture. Stuart progressed the session by drawing the bony points and muscles all over my legs. It took me a while to wash off my new tattoo but I'll never forget my first experience as a physio student, and how Stuart always taught us in a way that was interesting and easy to remember.

As physio students we all love learning about anatomy and practical aspects of the profession; after all what sort of physios will we become without an in depth knowledge of these things? BUT mention the words 'evidence based practice' or 'research' to us and watch our faces drop! This is how I came to be writing this foreword. When I again contacted Stuart for guidance, this time about a much-dreaded evidence based practice assignment, he kindly offered me the proofs to his new book to read and, well . . . here I am!

Finally the penny has dropped and it didn't take hours and hours of my time. I consider this book to be a student's best friend. It breaks down the concepts of research into appetizing bite sized pieces that I actually enjoyed consuming. It is written by someone who empathises with students regarding research and appreciates how complicated, confusing and (until understood) boring it can be. The book is very well structured, easy to follow and user friendly. Stuart highlights why so many of us dislike research, emphasises the importance of research to professionals, and puts it into perspective for students. He demonstrates how research can be a major aspect of healthcare where we as therapists can really make a difference (and isn't that what it's all about?)

The book includes interesting facts and useful tips throughout. It provides simple steps to approaching research, advice on how to organize your time and helps you understand what is expected of you as an undergraduate. Although it can't write your assignments for you . . . it will certainly help!

Stuart relates research to real life, helping us make research an intimate friend, rather than an abstract enemy. This book should help to stop you going round in circles, resolve any fears towards research, remove boredom and confusion, and even raise enthusiasm.

I dare you, after reading this book, not to find research just a little exciting and even start to ask and answer your own research questions. As we all know, research is an important part of making us effective physiotherapists and, therefore, I thank you Stuart for curing me of my research phobia and opening up a whole new exciting world to me which I never thought I'd dare to enter.

Rosie Hunt, 2008

He who asks a question is a fool for five minutes; he who does not ask a question remains a fool forever.

(Chinese Proverb)

Research means asking a question – it's as simple as that – well almost.

When I was a student, we didn't study research like many of today's students. I had to learn about research the hard way, ploughing my way through hundreds of articles, abstracts and methodological papers that may as well have been written in an alien language, which all had the effect of making me feel stupid – does that sound familiar?

Gradually, as my own research journey progressed, the mists cleared and I realised that research could be 'sexy' and 'exciting' but the books that I was reading did not seem to get this across, so I decided to write this book to prove that anyone can learn the basics of research methods, and that research is not something that you should be afraid of. All undergraduate students are introduced to research from a very early stage and unfortunately, many find the subject as baffling and frightening as I did.

This book is written for any student who feels that they are going round in confused circles, getting nowhere and losing the plot! This book provides students with the basic ammunition to get started on your project by learning about the processes of research and it helps you to avoid some of the pitfalls and dead-ends that affect students so often. It takes students from organising their thoughts, to choosing a topic, through to the production of a well-planned, ethical, methodologically sound and well-presented final report or dissertation.

It is written in plain language, uses real life examples and assumes no previous knowledge. It lets you painlessly into the baffling world of research methods.

Stuart Porter
March 2008

ACKNOWLEDGEMENTS

Once again, I am indebted to Elsevier for this opportunity, to Heidi Harrison, Siobhan Campbell and Veronika Krcilova. Claire Brown, Annabel Weaver, Susan Porter, Paul Edgar, Karen Edgar, Joe Woodcock, Marc Braid, Caroline Callister, Debbie Fagan. Ming Tham, Department of Chemical and Process Engineering, University of Newcastle upon Tyne, UK. Ronald J. Chenail, PhD co-editor, *The Qualitative Report*, Nova Southeastern University 3301, College Avenue, Fort Lauderdale, Florida, USA. L. W. Burts, NIH Contractor Customer Service, National Library of Medicine, 8600 Rockville Pike, Bethesda, MD, USA. Matt Holland and the Bournemouth University Library for permission to use their 'Citing References Guide'. Duncan James, Permissions Coordinator, John Wiley & Sons, Ltd., UK. June R. Levy, CINAHL Information Systems, 1509 Wilson Terrace, PO Box 871, Glendale, CA, USA. Dr Pauline Farren, Terri Lievesley. Jennifer Brown, Sandra Barton.

Thanks go to Matt Holland and the Bournemouth University Library, Dr Sally French, Freelance Researcher and Writer, Associate Lecturer at the Open University and Professor John Swain, Professor of Disability and Inclusion, Faculty of Health, Social Work and Education, University of Northumbria, Newcastle-upon-Tyne, UK for permission to reprint their work on how to write an academic assignment.

Dr Hugh Davies
Ethics and Training Advisor
Central Office for Research Ethics Committees
London, UK

Dr Bridget Dibb
Lecturer in Health Psychology
School of Health Professions and Rehabilitation Sciences
University of Southampton, UK

Maggie Donovan-Hall
Lecturer in Health Psychology
School of Health Professions and Rehabilitation Sciences
University of Southampton, UK

Mark Elkins BPhty, BA, MHSc, PhD
Co-Director
Centre for Evidence-Based Physiotherapy
Honorary Associate University of Sydney;
Research Physiotherapist
Respiratory Investigation Unit
Royal Prince Alfred Hospital
New South Wales,
Australia

Susan Porter RGN, DPSN
Senior Field Manager Innovex (UK) Ltd.

CHAPTER ONE

Making a start

Stuart Porter

STARTING YOUR RESEARCH JOURNEY

I run on the road, long before I dance under the lights
(Muhammad Ali)

If you are studying for a degree, at some point you are
going to start learning about research and research   **1**

methods. Research is as easy or as hard as you want to make it. One evening, when I was starting to plan this book, I asked my three daughters what they thought research was. Here are their comments:

(6 year old)
'I think research is about doing your best at work'

(9 year old)
'I think research means that you search for things on the web, say like you needed to find out something, you could do some research, and keep searching about it'

(10 year old)
'I think research is where you go over something over and over again, it is like revising I think'

These were interesting answers because:

1. They all came up with these definitions quickly, with no prompting.

2. All of their answers are different, for example although she did not realise it, my 6 year old had outlined the important link between research and clinical practice. My 9 year old had outlined the quest for knowledge and my 10 year old had expressed an embryonic opinion about academic rigour in research.

3. All of their answers have a positive theme (even though they have to live with the trials and tribulations of their father who is in the middle of his own PhD)!

Ask a typical undergraduate university student, however, and many of them have at best a dislike, and at worst, a hatred of learning about research methods. This is unfortunate, since without research of one form or another, we would probably still be living in caves. Incidentally, I then asked my children what they thought researchers looked like, their answers were: *'important, clever and hardworking'*!

Stop and think for a moment about your exposure to the word *research*, it is usually tagged on to the end of the national TV or radio news. Common examples of our exposure to the word *research* may include these two examples:

Scenario 1: An earth shattering finding of global importance, e.g. a new drug treatment for AIDS or a cure for cancer.

Scenario 2: A survey that has been carried out on the high street, e.g. where we are likely to go on holiday, or who we are likely to vote for in the next general election.

In Scenario 1, we tend to imagine people in white laboratory coats slaving away over a hot microscope, trying to make the world a better place. We also tend to

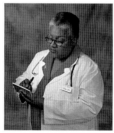

Fig. 1.1

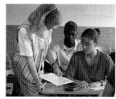

Fig. 1.2

think of these people as extremely clever, dedicated and infallible. In Scenario 2, we imagine a person with a clipboard on the high street and often perceive their behaviour as a nuisance or an intrusion. Research however, is much more than either of these.

SO WHY DO SO MANY STUDENTS DISLIKE RESEARCH?

If you like research and research methods, then I apologise, you can skip this section, if not read on. Most students do not like research, which is no great secret. Students are often introduced to research in the form of oddly titled modules or lectures with huge long words and concepts that are totally alien to them.

Lecturers spend a lot of time trying to make the subject as interesting as possible. I think that the reason behind this dislike is that students enter their degree course with a specific aim in mind, e.g. to become a physiotherapist, occupational therapist, nurse, doctor, etc. and then become a little disheartened when all this research methodology is thrown at them. Whether you like it or not however, research is now intimately bound to all health-related degree courses. Consider the example which follows.

WHY DO YOU NEED TO KNOW ABOUT RESEARCH?

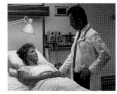

Example: You have a rare disease – let us call it Porter syndrome. You go to see Dr Smith.

Dr Smith has no interest in current research; he does what **Fig. 1.3** he has always done and gives you the tried and tested remedy of a sick note and antibiotics.

You now go to see Dr Jones, who learned about research methods while at university.

Dr Jones has done a search of the available research since the first time he saw you. He has performed a study of the most effective treatments for your disease and was able to assess which is the most likely to help you. He found a good study which suggests that antibiotics actually make Porter syndrome worse and the evidence suggests that the best treatment is with antiviral agents.

As a result:

1. You get better (always a bonus).

2. He publishes a case study about how he has helped you and this can now help future cases of Porter syndrome. *(Of course, there is no such syndrome as Porter syndrome – I just wanted the chance for something to be named after me!)*

So, which of these two doctors would you want to be treated by?

The box below gives some common thoughts that go through students' minds when they have to think about research.

'Nobody else seems to find research as difficult as I do'

'I want to be a clinician, not a researcher!'

'I am not clever enough to do research'

'I don't know where to start, it's all too overwhelming'

'I can't ask my supervisor that, they'll think that I'm stupid'

These feelings are common to all of us who have undertaken a research project. At the end of this chapter, we will return to these comments and then we can dismiss them once and for all.

MAKING RESEARCH A LITTLE LESS FRIGHTENING

The only thing we have to fear is fear itself

Franklin D. Roosevelt

WHO ARE RESEARCHERS?

Like most human fears, the fear of research is an irrational one and is probably based upon our preconceptions of what research is and what researchers are like. Research means asking a question and since this is something we all do every day, there is no logical reason for us to be afraid of the research process. Researchers are not locked away in laboratories experimenting with chemicals and test tubes, researchers are you and I. Read on to learn about some famous researchers.

Researchers have changed the world

Eratosthenes was the man who measured the world; he lived in Alexandria during the third century BC. He noticed that on the first day of summer in Syene (Egypt), the sun appeared directly overhead at noon and there were no shadows. At exactly the same time in Alexandria, however, the sun cast a shadow from a

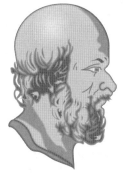

Fig. 1.4

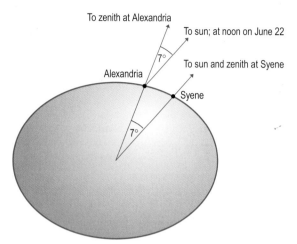

Fig. 1.5 Calculating Earth's circumference.

stick placed vertically; this meant that the earth could not be flat, as had always been thought.

Knowing the distance between Syene and Alexandria (he paid a man to pace out the distance between the two places) and assuming that the sun's rays were parallel when they struck the curved earth, he calculated the size of our planet using no more than two sticks and simple geometry. His result (about 25 000 miles for the circumference) proved remarkably accurate. He had no research grant, no ethical approval and no budget; he did all this with two wooden sticks.

Research lesson
Good research begins with a clear question and does not necessarily need a lot of equipment. In this case: I

believe that the world is not flat; I can not see the earth from above, so what is the next best method of measuring its curvature?

Researchers have also got it wrong

During a close approach by the planet Mars in 1877, an Italian astronomer thought he saw thin dark lines on the Martian surface. He called these lines 'channels', which in Italian is 'canali'. In Italian, 'canali' can mean either 'channels' or 'canals'. Somehow, the 'canal' version won out, implying that the lines were made by Martians.

The respected American astronomer, Percival Lowell, pounced on this story. He began to observe Mars through his powerful telescope and he too saw these canals, and insisted that they were real, going so far as to make up a whole Martian biology, describing a race of dying Martians that had to use these huge canals to carry water from the polar caps to their struggling cities and fields.

Lowell was an influential man in astronomy and he convinced other astronomers that these canals were real, despite the fact that very few astronomers reported actually seeing them. Lowell eventually mapped dozens of 'canals'. Lowell made many valuable contributions to the science of astronomy but unfortunately, when it came to Martian canals he was dead wrong, there are no canals on Mars, they were certainly of intelligent origin, but the intelligence was that of Percival Lowell. As late as the 1960s, maps of Mars featured these canals, when the robotic Mariner series of spacecraft flew past Mars, people on earth were surprised to learn that the canals did not exist and the maps of Mars had to be re-drawn.

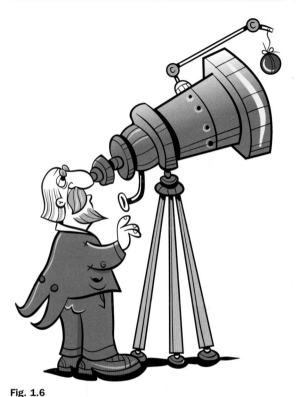

Fig. 1.6

Research lesson

Researchers are often tempted to see what they want to see. This is known as bias and we will discuss it later. For research to be good it must be methodical, use clear language, attempt to eliminate or at least acknowledge bias, and must not make unsupported claims. Lowell really wanted to believe that there were Martians and as well as convincing himself of this, he also convinced others of his research findings – from a flawed first step in his research, he took a step too far.

Observation: I cannot really see anything on Mars.
Research finding: A race of dying Martians.

There are accepted rules and procedures for carrying out research. While these are apparently complex and often confusing, they are very important to ensure that all research is ethical, moral and accurate.

GETTING STARTED ON YOUR RESEARCH – THE HARD PART

The beginning is the most important part of the work

Plato

Students often spend many months seemingly going round in circles and becoming more and more distressed as the deadline for the submission of their project or dissertation approaches. Most supervisors are experienced enough to recognise this and are able to steer the student along a path that will help.

It is worth remembering at this point that you have *not* been going round in circles and you *probably have* been thinking (albeit subconsciously) about what you want to do. The role of the next few pages is to help you to capture the area of interest and start to focus it into a workable project.

Pick a topic that interests you

Students often state that they have no idea what they want to do for their research project; everybody however, has something that they are interested in, and that is the logical place to start. Often all that is needed is a person – usually your supervisor – to help you think things through logically, and help you to define, and refine your area of interest.

As the deadline approaches it is tempting to pick the first subject that pops into your head. The best advice at this stage is do not panic, and ensure that the project that you do choose is your own project and not someone else's. You will be spending a lot of time on this and you need to make the process as enjoyable and smooth as possible – this is of course more likely if you are interested in what you are doing.

 STUDENT TIP In the early stages keep a notepad with you for when ideas pop into your head – otherwise they are likely to pop out of your head again.

BEING A RESEARCH STUDENT AND USING YOUR SUPERVISOR

Often the time allocated to you to complete an under-graduate research project is very limited and many students make the mistake of choosing a project that is too ambitious. This results in a project which is incomplete and can be easily criticised by the marker. A later chapter will discuss what your markers are looking for. At undergraduate level, examiners are usually more interested in your ability to follow the research process accurately; it is often acceptable to repeat an existing piece of research or repeat a project but on a different population. In some respects, the choice of topic is not as important as how you address the question. You are not expected at undergraduate level to add to the body of existing academic knowledge; in fact this is one of the definitions of a PhD, and most PhDs take a minimum of 3 years' full-time study or 5–6 years' part-time study.

If you go into your undergraduate project aiming to discover something completely new, you will run into major problems.

 STUDENT TIP Supervisors were once students, and they do know what you are going through.

When you reach the point that you are ready to commence your research project, you will usually be assigned a supervisor. This will often be a member of teaching staff that you already know, or, in the case of a higher degree such as a PhD, you may have a team of people who come in and out of the project at various times according to their expertise. Maintaining a good working relationship with you supervisor is like any partnership; it takes work and constant two-way communication.

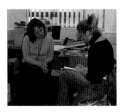

Fig. 1.7 The life of a research supervisor (with thanks to Dr Pauline Farren and Terri Lievesley).

It may not seem so, but your supervisors probably have more pressure on them than you. Supervisors are often expected to carry a full teaching load; complete their own research projects or PhDs; publish; and act as a shoulder to cry on for their students, children, husbands/wives, etc. Deep down, students know this and do not like to bother their supervisors with what they feel are silly questions, but in the case of the research student–supervisor relationship, a lack of communication can be disastrous.

 STUDENT TIP   Students who tend to do best are the ones that communicate with their supervisors.

Check your university rules and regulations about supervision, but here are some general points worth considering:

1. The supervisor is as busy as you are.

2. The supervisor is probably under more pressure than you are.

3. Supervisors are not perfect, and they will not know everything about the area that you are researching; what they can do, however, is comment on the process, rigour, project design and steps that you need to follow.

4. The amount of time that the supervisor can spend with you will be limited. Prepare in advance of any meetings you have. If you have not done any work since your last meeting, cancel the next one and rearrange the meeting

for when you have something more to discuss.

5. Adhere to any agreed deadlines. This means that you need to make sure that the deadlines you jointly set are always realistic; the supervisor will not mind if you are honest about this.

6. Be honest with your supervisor at all times. If you do not understand something that they have said or asked you to do – you must make this clear – do not sit and nod, as the supervisor will then naturally assume that you fully understand.

7. Communicate with your supervisor little and often. In the age of e-mail, there is no excuse for this not happening.

8. Remember that the supervisor cannot rewrite the project for you and there will probably be a cut-off point at which they are not allowed to comment on your work. Some universities may have regulations that forbid them from looking at completed drafts of your report, so do not take offence if the supervisor states that they are unable to look at your work.

9. Take a notebook with you and make notes as you talk. The supervisor may let you tape-record the conversation but you will need to gain permission before doing this. If you cannot make notes during the meeting, write down the main points of the discussion immediately afterwards.

10. Acknowledge your supervisors in your final report, and write them a thank you letter afterwards.

Form 1.1 shows a simple format that you might find useful to record meetings with your supervisor.

Student's Name	Date	Supervisor

Project Title
Summary of Points Discussed
Action by Student
Action by Supervisor(s)
Date of Next Meeting

Form 1.1   Research student/supervisor meeting record.

WHAT TO DO WHEN THINGS GO WRONG

Occasionally, the relationship between you and your supervisor may break down. If you sense that this is happening, the best advice is to seek a meeting with them rather than letting things escalate. If this still does not work you will need to change supervisors but do this in a manner that is professional and does not annoy your other academic lecturers.

DEVELOPING YOUR IDEA FOR A RESEARCH PROJECT

You will probably have some idea about what research area you want to look at. Let us compare this to a large lump of dough; it is a bit sticky and difficult to see anything inside clearly enough to make a research project and so it needs to be refined and worked into a suitable project (Fig. 1.8).

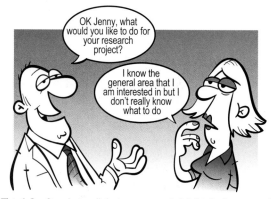

Fig. 1.8 Opening a dialogue – an early joint role for you and your supervisor.

The next phase involves kneading this doughy idea and refining it into a workable project. Think of this process as squeezing your idea through a funnel – this is not as easy as it sounds – do not underestimate the length of time that this apparently simple process can take (Fig. 1.9). After all, dough, like your early research idea, is still likely to be sticky.

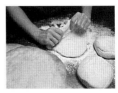

Fig. 1.9

We can now look at this process in a little more detail and start to think about the nature of the project you are interested in. Now imagine squeezing your research idea through the funnel again, but now start to think about what you hope to come out of the other end of the funnel, i.e. what are you really interested in (Fig. 1.10)? We do not yet need to start worrying about methods; at this stage what we need is a clear question. Let us assume that your general area of interest is back pain; that is the first step. The next step is to think about which aspects of back pain in particular you want to enquire about.

Look at Figure 1.11 and notice how the choice of your research question dictates the method that you will eventually use, not the other way around. Students often make the mistake of first of all choosing a method, e.g. 'I want to do a questionnaire' and then try to think of a question to fit.

By this stage you are now able to decide whether you should be looking towards a quantitative or qualitative study. Later chapters cover these in more detail but for now here is an introduction to these two types of research (Table 1.1).

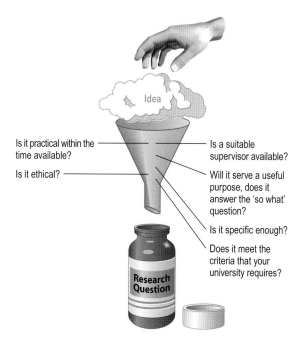

Is it practical within the time available?

Is it ethical?

Is a suitable supervisor available?

Will it serve a useful purpose, does it answer the 'so what' question?

Is it specific enough?

Does it meet the criteria that your university requires?

Research Question

Fig. 1.10

WHAT MAKES A GOOD RESEARCH QUESTION?

To be or not to be, is that a research question?

(with apologies to Shakespeare)

A good research question should:

■ Address a real need or problem
■ Be researchable, i.e. 'do-able' given your time and other constraints

I am interested in doing a project on back pain

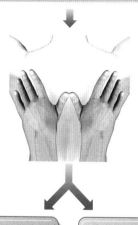

I am interested in looking at what it is really like living with back pain and what effect it has on people's lives.

I am interested in looking at the levels of pain that people with back pain experience.

If we are interested in examining feelings, perspectives or patients and attitudes then this will usually lead to a qualitative study.

If we want to quantify something, i.e. put a figure on it, this will lead to a quantitative study.

Fig. 1.11

TABLE 1.1   COMMON FEATURES OF QUALITATIVE AND QUANTITATIVE RESEARCH

Qualitative	Quantitative
The aim of qualitative analysis is a complete, detailed description of a topic.	In quantitative research, we count features and construct statistical models in an attempt to explain what we observe.
The researcher may only have a broad impression of what may arise.	The researcher knows clearly in advance what he/she is looking for.
The design emerges as the study unfolds.	All aspects of the study are carefully pre-designed before data collection commences.
The researcher is the data-gathering instrument.	The researcher uses tools, such as questionnaires, to collect numerical data.
Data tend to be in the form of words, pictures or objects.	Data are in the form of numbers and statistics.
Qualitative data are more 'rich', time consuming, and less able to be generalised.	Quantitative data are more efficient, and able to test hypotheses.
The researcher tends to become subjectively immersed in the subject matter.	The researcher strives to remain distanced from the subject matter.

- Inspire your interest and keep you interested for the length of the study
- Should not be so general that it needs to be split into many smaller questions
- Should not be so narrow that it is not likely to be useful to anyone.

TEST YOURSELF ON RESEARCH IDEAS

There follows here four ideas, all of which have a flaw of some kind. Read them and see if you can work out what the problem of each is before looking below at the answers.

1. I would like to do a project that will make the world a better place.

2. I would like to do a questionnaire on something.

3. I want to find out what type of injuries children who are physically abused suffer.

4. I am interested in doing a research project that looks at how quickly people regain knee flexion after knee surgery.

Answers

1. Much too broad, not specific, not measurable (not SMART).

2. In this case, the student has put the cart before the horse; they have a method without a question. You should work on your research question first of all, then decide on the most appropriate research tool.

3. Interesting subject but ethically very difficult and not practical if you are an undergraduate.

Continued

4. Too many hidden or confounding variables, e.g. what exactly do you mean by knee surgery; how long are you going to measure for; what drugs are the patients on, etc.

More about your research question

The earlier quote from Plato stated that the beginning was the most important part of the work. This is certainly true when you are planning a research project. Get the beginning right and the project gains momentum as you progress and becomes an enjoyable part of your studies; get the beginning wrong and you run the risk of having to backtrack at a later date, at a time when you have no time left!

Research is sometimes referred to as a journey. Like any journey, there is usually more than one way to reach your destination. Each way has advantages and disadvantages but one thing is certain, you are more likely to successfully arrive at your destination if you know exactly what form of transport you are going to take; the pros and cons of each method and that you are confident that this form of transport will safely get you to your destination. There is often no right or wrong way to undertake a project in the same way that a train is not necessarily right and a bus wrong, and as your choice of transport depends on various complex factors, so does your choice of research method.

You may find this analogy helpful when planning your research. You can take a train or a bus to get to the university in the same way that you can use a quantitative or qualitative approach to address a research problem, and in the same way that the journey on the

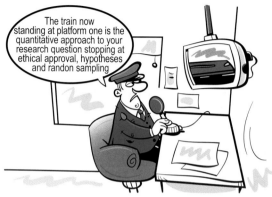

Fig. 1.12

bus and the train will be different, the quantitative and qualitative approaches will also give you different perspectives on your topic. The problem starts when you get on the bus and you are not sure of your destination – in some cases this is acceptable, e.g. some qualitative research does not have pre-existing hypotheses and actually generates theory as it goes along. This is a fascinating aspect of qualitative research and is a little like trying to lay the tracks a few yards ahead for the train you are travelling on; the danger here is that a student may lay the tracks in the wrong direction.

Above all, you will be helped if you have a clear destination in mind. Think about it as though you are walking into a busy airport or train station. What you need is a clear indication of what time the train or plane sets off, where it is going and what you will need to accomplish the journey. In research terms, this means in order to make your academic life as safe as possible, you should have a clear title and from this point on, you should know your destination. (This does not mean that you should know in advance what the results are going to be. It means that you have a clear strategy for how to get to the results and you know why you have taken the approach that you have done.) If you can maintain this focus (not narrow-mindedness) throughout your research project then you are likely to be much 'safer' in academic terms (Table 1.2).

TABLE 1.2 DIFFERENT APPROACHES AND THE PHILOSOPHY BEHIND THEM	
Ask yourself this question	**The research train for comparison**
Are you sure that you have chosen the correct research method?	In other words, are you sure you want the train?
Are you sure that you have accurately outlined your methodological stance?	In other words, are you sure you are on the right train?
Have you started your protocol and opened discussions with your supervisor?	In other words, have you bought a ticket?
Do you know what your university's guidelines are? Fail to follow these and you risk failing the project.	In other words, have you paid? Fail to pay and you will be thrown off the train.
How will you know when you have completed your project?	In other words, do you know when to get off the train?

CHOOSING A TOPIC

We will now go back to the start of our research project, which is – choosing a topic. This subject is so important that we are going to spend some more time discussing problems and pitfalls.

Problem: The student who picks a topic which is too broad

'I would like to do some research into levels of pain, stiffness and function after shoulder replacement and I want to give all my patients a questionnaire followed by an interview and then measure their range of movement 1 month after their operation'

This is admirable but a little dangerous. Let us say that you have 6 months to plan and undertake your project – now, if I tell you that my own PhD, which has taken 6 years of dedication and hard work has added a small fraction to what we already know about how people exercise for ankylosing spondylitis and can largely be summarised on a piece of A4 – that should tell you about how limited your time is.

Solution

As a rule it is a good idea to pick something that is narrow, do it well and include only one variable. For example, do not set out to look at pain, range of movement and function after total shoulder replacement, instead pick one, such as movement, acknowledging the limitations of the study, and suggest that you will look at the other parameters of pain and function in the future.

This means that your whole project can maintain focus and have a consistent thread and as a result, it is less likely to be shot full of holes on submission.

Problem: The student who picks something that they cannot do

'I want to create a questionnaire about depression among nursing students because it's never been done before'

Occasionally students pick topics that they cannot do. For example, you wish to undertake a piece of complex gait analysis but you have never spent any time in a gait laboratory. Another common example is that a student will pick a research method that they perceive to be an easy option, not realising that this is not the case. Typically, this involves giving a questionnaire to participants without realising that the design of the questionnaire is not adequate and that the questionnaire has not been validated. The supervisor should pick up on these problems at an early stage.

Solution

The remedy for these involves some hard thinking about why you have chosen to undertake this project. It is better to simplify and get it right than to drown early on.

Problem: The student who picks a research subject that is too detached from reality

'I want to do a survey of the colour of medicine bottles in Antarctica'

Students sometimes pick a topic that is so abstract that it is difficult to see the relevance of the results to anybody in the future.

Solution

If you think that this is the case for your idea, then you need to speak very carefully with your supervisor to check that you will not be penalised for the project not having any clinical usefulness. However, it is probably harder to get the interest of the reader and a good mark if the project is about the colour of medicine bottles in Antarctica! Having said that, at undergraduate level, the emphasis is on the process that you have followed rather than the actual topic. If you can construct an argument that there might be a placebo effect to the colour of medicine bottles with clinical implications, then it may be valid to do the study.

Problem: The student who does somebody else's idea

'My supervisor wants me to help him out with his own research, which has something to do with bronchitis'

Solution

If you are interested in the area then fine, go ahead.

If you are not particularly interested, then you need to make this clear; the supervisor should not mind.

Problem: The student who has no idea what topic to choose

'I've got no idea what I'm going to do'

Solution

Read this chapter from the beginning again . . .

PLANNING AND MANAGING YOUR TIME

There are many useful books available on time management, the problem is that we usually do not have time to read them.

Students often postpone their research until the last minute, sometimes for sound reasons – but do not forget that even an elephant looks small when it is a long way off, and as it gets closer it is liable to crush you!

The only way to be successful with study is to take a long-term view and find a strategy that works for you. You can also find useful information in the Study Skills department of your university or college library. Many people find a Gantt chart useful. It permits you to plan out a timeline and you can cross off items as you successfully complete them. Fig. 1.14 gives an example of a simple Gantt chart.

Now we will return to the statements that we introduced near the start of this chapter and note the answers.

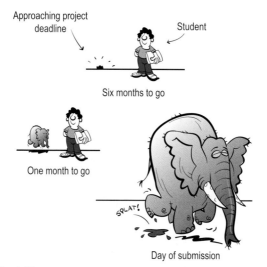

Fig. 1.13

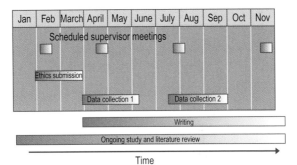

Fig. 1.14 A simple Gantt chart.

'Nobody else seems to find research as difficult as I do'

– Oh, yes they do. It is not easy and like most things in life it looks easy when you speak to somebody who has already done it.

'I want to be a clinician, not a researcher!'

– In the twenty-first century, it is not possible to be a clinician and not embrace research. Put simply, your patients deserve to know what works and what does not, and that your treatments are based upon the best available evidence.

'I am not clever enough to do research'

– Yes you are, research is as simple or as complicated as you want to make it.

'I don't know where to start, it's all too overwhelming'

– Read this chapter again. Make small deliberate moves into your project, stay focussed and use the experience of your supervisor.

> *'I can't ask my supervisor that, they'll think that I'm
> stupid'*
>
> – No they will not, or at least they should not if they
>   are good supervisors. They are more likely to think
>   you are stupid if you never ask them anything until
>   it is too late, e.g. 1 week before your project is
>   due to be submitted!

SUMMARY

1. Don't be afraid – research is as easy or as hard as you want to make it.
2. Your research is unlikely to be perfect – acknowledge this.
3. Chose a topic area in which you are interested.
4. Use your supervisor.
5. Start with a broad aim and narrow it down.
6. Make sure that you stick to the aim.
7. Think carefully about what you are trying to achieve.
8. Have a clear train of thought and do not get distracted unless you know you are going wrong.
9. Make sure you have a basic understanding of the method that you have chosen and what it can and cannot do for you.
10. Plan your time so that you can take your time.

CONCLUSION

Once you have got a research idea that follows the university guidelines and with which you and your supervisor are happy, this is the time to stop reflecting and asking other armchair experts who delight in suggesting changes – I promise you, taking notice of those will backfire at worst and at best will only slow you down. Trust in yourself and your supervisor to know best.

You now need to move on and concentrate on thinking about the nuts and bolts of your project. These are discussed in the following chapters.

LEARNING OUTCOMES

After reading this chapter you should have a basic understanding of . . .

- How to start your research journey
- Why students do not like research
- Why you need to know about research
- Making research a little less frightening
- Famous researchers
- Getting started – the hard part
- The responsibilities of being a student and a supervisor
- How to use your supervisor
- What to do when things go wrong
- How to develop your research idea
- Common features of qualitative and quantitative research
- What makes a good research question
- Problems and pitfalls
- Organising your time.

CHAPTER TWO

The researcher's view of the world: research paradigms

Stuart Porter

Is all that we see or seem but a dream within a dream?

(Edgar Allan Poe)

Researchers try to discover the truth, but what is truth? This short chapter introduces you to a potentially difficult but important subject, and although at first, this chapter may seem abstract, the subject of what we can and cannot know, our views of how the world works and the nature of reality is a fundamental part of research methods.

What do you see here (Fig. 2.1), a wine glass or two people facing each other? If you look at this picture for long enough, your brain will begin switching between the two images in an attempt to work out which one is 'true' – in fact both are true – as a research student you should acknowledge the fact that there is more than one way to view the world around us.

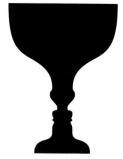

Fig. 2.1

WHAT IS A PARADIGM?

Human behaviour, our ability to ask questions and therefore undertake research is based upon our beliefs about how things work, and these beliefs are in turn shaped by our culture, education, and life experiences. While some schools of research take the view that the world is measurable and quantifiable, others believe that things are not quite so simple. These 'world views' are more accurately known as paradigms.

A paradigm is a set of assumptions and values that makes up a way of viewing reality for the community that shares them. There are various paradigms but the simplest way to divide them is into positivist and naturalist paradigms.

PARADIGM SHIFTS

From time to time in our history, we totally rethink our views of the world – this is known as a paradigm shift.

Throughout most of the world's history we believed that the world was flat – but now we know that is it round – or at least we have been *told* that it is round

(Fig. 2.2). Even though you have probably not seen the earth from space, you accept this as 'truth' and you would be laughed at if you suggested otherwise. There is an overwhelming collective body of knowledge and experts telling us that the world is round, much in the same way as that 500 years ago, when there were similar experts telling us that it was actually flat.

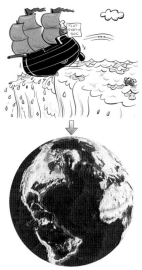

Or, here is an example from the world of medicine (Fig. 2.3).

Fig. 2.2

In the Middle Ages, a headache was likely to be blamed on an evil spirit, since this was part of the accepted culture; this did not seem odd at all and would have been readily accepted. You would have been laughed at if you had suggested that a tumour could have caused a headache. Nowadays, you would be in a minority in suggesting the evil spirit hypothesis.

Medicine in the twentieth century was geared towards looking for organic causes of disease rather than spiritual, although in recent years, there has been an upsurge in alternative medicine and non-traditional methods of healing – we live in interesting times of multiple paradigms.

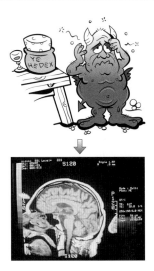

Fig. 2.3

WHAT CAN A RESEARCHER LEARN ABOUT THE WORLD?

Research, like most things in life, is complex. A good example of this can be taken from the world of physics. Physicists were traditionally embedded in a world of certainty, equations and hard fact (the quantitative or positivist paradigm), until a scientist named Werner Heisenberg came up with a radical proposal. Heisenberg had a shocking but clear realisation about the limits of physical knowledge: the act of observing alters the reality being observed. This would come to be known as the uncertainty principle. To measure the properties of a particle, such as an electron, one needs to use a measuring device, usually light or radiation. But the energy in this radiation affects the particle being observed. This led to the belief that the very act of measuring something changes its behaviour; this is central to all research.

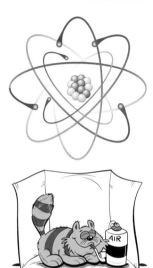

Schrödinger's cat (Fig. 2.4) is another famous illustration proposed by Erwin Schrödinger in 1935. It serves to demonstrate the apparent conflict between what the truth is and what reality is. It is

Fig. 2.4

as follows (simplified): Place a living cat into a box and close the lid; according to quantum physics, the cat is both simultaneously dead and alive. It is only when the researcher opens the box and inspects the condition of the cat that this state is lost, and the cat becomes one or the other (dead or alive). This situation is called *quantum indeterminacy* or *the observer's paradox*: the observation or measurement itself affects an outcome, so that it can never be known what the outcome would have been if it were not observed. So in research terms, as soon as we undertake a research intervention we automatically change our environment for better or for worse.

Changing reality without realising it: the Hawthorne effect

To further complicate matters, there is a concept known as the Hawthorne effect. This means that human behaviour may be altered simply because a person knows that they are being researched. This was first identified in a research project in the 1920s and 1930s at the Hawthorne Plant of the Western Electric Company in Illinois, USA. Researchers examined the physical and environmental influences on the workplace (e.g. brightness of lights, humidity) and later, moved into the psychological aspects (e.g. tea breaks, group pressure, working hours, managerial leadership).

The key finding of the study was that regardless of whatever area the researchers changed (in research language this is known as manipulation of variables), the productivity of the workers improved. Possibly the workers were pleased to receive the attention from the researchers who expressed an interest in them. This is important to us as therapists. Consider a patient who has been having a treatment for 6 months which has been unsuccessful. If he is referred to a different therapist who changes the treatment, it is likely to have a positive benefit, simply owing to the Hawthorne effect. Indeed, in my own clinical experience, it was always much easier to get positive results when treatment was changed from a previously unsuccessful one – and not because I was a particularly great physiotherapist. Now do you see why knowledge of research methods is important to you as a therapist or healthcare practitioner?

We will look at two example projects; one quantitative and one qualitative.

1. We will look at an experiment to assess a person's posture using video analysis.
   Now, as soon as you mention that you are researching posture, people stand up straight – so right away you are not measuring their true posture, you are measuring this newly adopted posture instead.

2. We will do a focus group that enquires about attitudes towards group exercise.
   You are probably going to get more favourable answers from the people that volunteered for the focus group in the first place, because they like attending groups. Then, when you do the focus group itself, the people who are in attendance are likely to behave more positively, because they know that you are observing them and in particular their reaction to group work.

Practical example

You want to undertake a research study investigating student's opinions about some recent exams that they have taken. You decide to undertake a focus group to assess the 'truth' about what the students really think about these exams.

What might influence the data (truth) that you obtain?

Think about the following scenarios:

Scenario 1: If the students have already had their exams marked

Scenario 2: If the exams have not yet been marked

Scenario 3: If the student has passed the exams and knows this

Scenario 4: If the student has failed and the researcher was also their examiner

Scenario 5: If the student still has more exams to come

Scenario 6: Are students likely to behave in the same way in a tape-recorded interview with a lecturer present as they would if chatting in the pub with each other?

Some suggested answers to these scenarios:

1. The student will no longer feel under pressure to 'play the game,' you may get more honest answers from a student who has no hidden agenda than if the student still had their exam to sit.

2. The student may be exceptionally kind in the hope that this will influence the lecturer who is about to mark the exam. Alternatively, they may be so nervous about their forthcoming exams that they act out of character or are even hostile towards the researcher.

3. This student will certainly be more relaxed, which may encourage them to act more honestly and openly.

4. The student may have an 'axe to grind' and, as a result, be overly negative. This may be seen as a chance for them to 'get their own back', or it may be a genuine belief on their part (we are back to multiple realities again).

5. The student may not attend the focus group at all, or may subconsciously believe that by attending

the group, they are showing a mature willing attitude to the person who is about to examine them in the future.

6. In a word – 'No'. The responses will not be the same. The social dynamics of students in a pub are not the same as the student talking to a lecturer; in the latter, there are things such as professionalism, power differentials, the need to act in a certain way in front of your lecturer, etc. If you are going to tape-record the interview, as a researcher you will need to make it clear to the participants that you will not identify them personally from anything that they might say – a later chapter on ethics discusses this.

From the relatively simple example above, we have generated multiple realities and many complex factors that could influence the data that the researcher obtains. Now imagine how much more complex and difficult it would be to manage this project if we were doing a focus group about drug abuse, euthanasia, abortion, or some other sensitive topic.

THE RELEVANCE OF PARADIGMS TO YOUR RESEARCH PROJECT

No knowledge is complete or perfect

Carl Sagan

The word 'thesis' derives from the Greek word for 'position'. Whenever you undertake a piece of research, you must acknowledge from which paradigm you are working, and the position of your thesis. It is important at any level to recognise that no single stance is perfect.

Higher level students such as PhDs often devote large numbers of pages to these philosophical arguments; at undergraduate level it is probably not so important but nonetheless, a grasp of this topic can only serve to impress your reader (or marker). A well written project will contain a section that clearly illustrates the stance of the writer, and an acknowledgement of the limitations and strengths of this stance.

Paradigms provide the foundations for conducting research and provide the researcher with a platform from which to interpret the world (Morgan 1983). The positivist paradigm assumes a world of objects, objectivity and assumptions which can be measured independently of one another. This type of research portrays truth as a single, measurable reality. Positivist researchers stand at a distance from their subjects and maintain that the knower can be distinguished from the known.

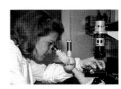

Fig. 2.5

The qualitative paradigm attempts to understand the world from the viewpoint of its participants (note the use of the word participants rather than subjects in qualitative research) through detailed

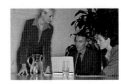

Fig. 2.6

portrayals and description of the richness associated with human behaviour (Wildemuth 1993). This paradigm rejects a cause-and-effect construct and the separation between researcher and respondent is less clear.

TABLE 2.1   POSITIVIST AND NATURALIST PARADIGMS COMPARED

Belief about	Positivist paradigm (quantitative)	Naturalist paradigm (qualitative)
The nature of reality	Reality is single	Realities are multiple
The relationship of knower to the known	Knower and known are independent of each other	The knower and the known interact and are inseparable
The possibility of generalisation	Time- and context-free generalisations can be made	Only time- and context-bound working hypotheses can be made
The role of values	Inquiry is value-free	Inquiry is value-bound

The strengths and weaknesses of qualitative and quantitative research have been a hot debate for many years, especially in the social sciences: the so-called 'paradigm war' (Fig. 2.7).

Occasionally, you may encounter people who argue with you that quantitative research is better then qualitative research or vice versa. This is naïve, since they are totally different types of research. If you want to ascribe figures to a project and look for a cause-and-effect relationship, you need to go down the quantitative route, whereas if you are interested in exploring a topic and delving in to the 'why' then this lends itself to a qualitative project. If you do come across such an argument, ask the person this question:

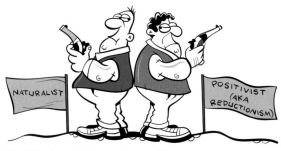

Fig. 2.7   Opposing research paradigms.

If you are stranded on a desert island, which is the most useful, a torch or an apple?

They will probably look at you as if you are mad and say something like 'it depends' and they would be quite right,

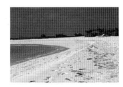

Fig. 2.8

it is a silly question, since the correct answer depends on what you need. If you are starving to death you need an apple, but if you can see a ship in the distance you need a torch. So in the same way, qualitative and quantitative research are different.

Epistemology

The branch of philosophy that studies the nature of knowledge, its presuppositions and foundations and its extent and validity is known as epistemology. This word refers to our theory of knowledge, in particular how we acquire knowledge. How do we really know what we know? The solution has been for humans to define knowledge in an alternative fashion, one where knowledge can only be 'asserted'. Knowledge is therefore not conditional; it is a convention of society. A number of writers have proposed the need to change our concept of science. Some have suggested that science may be more appropriately described in terms of problem- or puzzle-solving.

Ontology
This word has a long history in philosophy, in which it refers to the subject of existence. An ontology is a set of concepts, such as things or events that are specified in some way.

PULLING IT ALL TOGETHER
When you are discussing or writing up your research project, it will impress the reader if you pay some attention to the concept of paradigms and try to get across to the reader, the philosophical arguments for what you have done (the methodological issues); why you chose to do it that particular way; and the benefits and limitations of the method that you have chosen. These are important arguments that are closely linked to paradigms.

If you stop and think about the nature of the project that you are doing, and the things that might affect the truth of the results, then you will generate a much more coherent research project and your overall research experience will be more enjoyable.

Ask yourself . . .
Ask yourself the questions in Figure 2.9 before you put pen to paper.

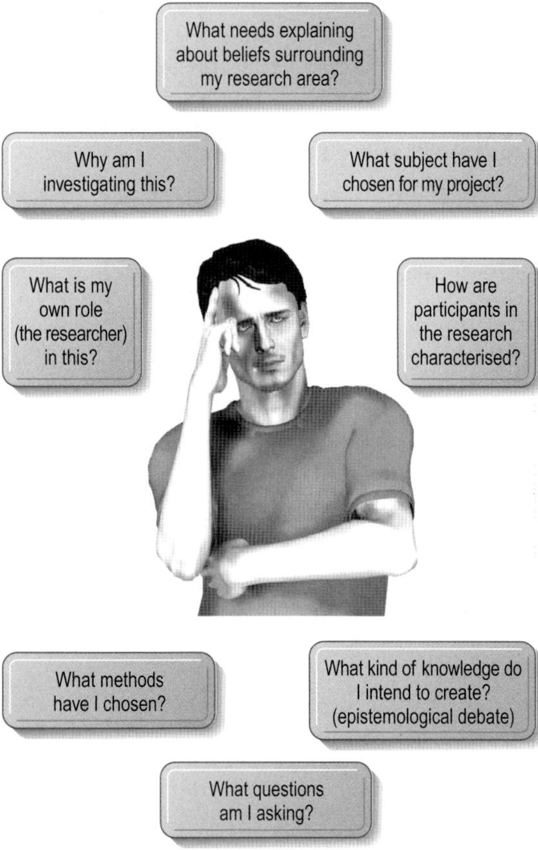

Fig. 2.9 Ask yourself . . .

SUMMARY

1. There are various 'camps' or research paradigms. You need to base yourself in the one which will best answer your research question.
2. Try to grasp the concept of paradigms and make some reference to them when writing up your research.
3. Each paradigm has a different view of things, not necessarily better or worse, just different.
4. Do not get drawn into a paradigm war.
5. Always choose the right research tool for the right job.
6. The very act of doing research may change your results.

LEARNING OUTCOMES

After reading this chapter you should have a basic understanding of . . .
- What a paradigm is
- Paradigm shifts
- What researchers can learn about the world
- The relevance of paradigms and your research project
- Positivist and naturalist paradigms compared.

REFERENCES

Morgan G 1983 Research strategies: Modes of engagement. In: Morgan G (ed.) Beyond method. SAGE, Beverly Hills, CA.

Wildemuth B 1993 Post-positivist research: two examples of methodological pluralism. Library Quarterly 63:450–468.

CHAPTER THREE

Literature review and essay writing

Stuart Porter

If you believe everything you read, better not read
(Japanese proverb)

The thought of writing a literature review fills many students with dread. This chapter will give you some suggestions to make the process a little less daunting.

WHAT IS A LITERATURE REVIEW?
A literature review is an account of what has been published on a topic in the past by researchers. Its purpose **49**

is to convey to the reader what has been established about a topic, and what the strengths and weaknesses of each finding are. A literature review must be defined by a guiding concept and it should not just be a list of all of the material that you can find, or a collection of summaries. The person reading your literature review will probably be looking for your competence in the following areas:

1. The ability to follow the guidelines given to you.
2. The ability to scan the literature efficiently to identify a set of useful articles and books.
3. The ability to use your knowledge of the research process to identify 'good research', i.e. unbiased and valid studies.
4. The ability to put all of the information together in a flowing logical and appropriate style.

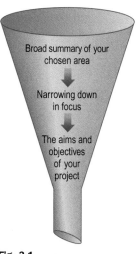

Broad summary of your chosen area

↓

Narrowing down in focus

↓

The aims and objectives of your project

In Chapter 1, we used the analogy of a funnel to focus our research question. We can again use a funnel (Fig. 3.1) to describe the shape of a good literature review, i.e. broad at the top but quickly narrowing down to a point. The literature review is your best opportunity to grab the attention of the reader and

Fig. 3.1

to make them want to read on; unfortunately this opportunity is often wasted and reading student literature reviews can be a painful experience.

You may find a mindmap useful. For example, Figure 3.2 is a hypothetical mindmap for a review on stroke.

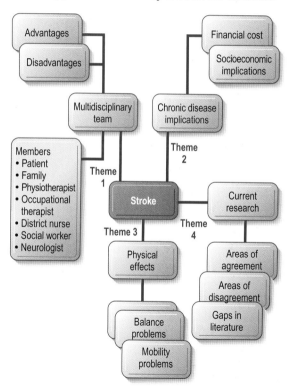

Fig. 3.2 A hypothetical mindmap.

BACKING UP YOUR ARGUMENTS

When you write a piece of academic work you must always acknowledge where the idea came from. There are two ways that you can to this: you can either quote the author directly or you can paraphrase but in both cases you have to acknowledge the original source. This is known as referencing and is always a cause of great confusion among students. There are different styles of referencing but the Harvard system is commonly used in the UK.

QUALITIES OF A GOOD LITERATURE REVIEW

See Figure 3.3.

Ask yourself the following questions when you are writing a literature review

How many words am I permitted?

–   You need to work out how many words you are going to devote to each aspect of your literature review; this can be rough in the early stages but you do need to bear this in mind. If your literature review is relatively short, you will need to narrow down the focus quite quickly, if you go over the word limit you may be penalised.

What research question do I want to guide the reader towards?

–   Do not simply launch into a stream of information. Explain why the topic is important and give the reader an idea of where you are going in your literature review. Readers like to feel reassured that they know what to expect. Then

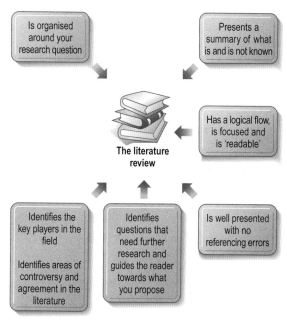

Fig. 3.3

review the literature, organising it in a clear and easy to follow manner. You do not have to include every study that has ever been conducted on your subject; only the ones that are most important to what you want to say. After you have introduced your topic, reviewed the literature and written a conclusion, you then need to include a reference list at the end of your paper.

What is the scope of my literature review and is it logically organised?

–   Do not make the job of reading it harder than it needs to be. In which ever way you proceed, you will need a plan. For example, you may wish to organise the review chronologically, or as it relates to different perspectives on an issue or to opposing views of a research area.

What types of publications am I using and more importantly, what is their academic credibility?

–   Check the guidelines about what are acceptable sources of information for your project. The internet is certainly one of the great inventions of our time but not so when it comes to writing literature reviews; going online to search for research is like trying to fill a glass with water from Niagara Falls. If you simply go on to the internet you are likely to end-up with thousands of references to your topic, many of which will not be quality controlled and may be easily criticised by your marker; this does not apply to searching recognised databases, which are discussed later. Remember the concept of peer review and journal impact factors.

Who and what are the key researchers/theories in the field?

–   As you continue your search through your chosen topic you should start to see familiar names. These are the key contributors in the field, it would be

very unwise not to make mention of these
authors.

Has my search been wide enough to ensure that all the
key articles are included, and has it been narrow enough
to exclude any irrelevant material?

– Let us assume that you want to look for articles
about the effects of group exercise for people with
arthritis of the knee, and you go onto a search
engine such as MEDLINE and type in 'exercise'.
Databases such as MEDLINE are excellent but the
MEDLINE computer will not know exactly which
articles you are looking for, so it will do exactly
what you requested and it will give you every
article with 'exercise' in its title. This could mean
exercise in the context of cardiac rehabilitation,
antenatal classes, sport, back pain and so on.
Table 3.1 illustrates this.

Look at Table 3.1 and note how the more specific
you are, the more specific the articles will be (and

TABLE 3.1 NUMBER OF CITATIONS RETRIEVED VIA MEDLINE ON 26 SEPTEMBER 2005	
Term typed	Number of articles retrieved
'Exercise'	135 343
'Exercise' and 'knee'	3024
'Exercise' and 'knee' and 'osteoarthritis'	222
'Exercise' and 'knee' and 'osteoarthritis' and 'group'	78

more manageable in number). The risk here is that you may omit wider searches that may have been relevant to your project, so for example, if you are conducting a literature review on group exercise for knee pain in arthritis, you may also want to search under psychological implications of arthritis, and financial implications of group exercise, to broaden your literature review. Which topics you do and do not need to search under will be dictated by your original project aims or the original research question. This is why your ability to choose a research question and stick with it is so important. If your project only wishes to look at pain levels, then there is no point in searching under the financial implications, but if you are interested in a different aspect of group exercise, e.g. why patients choose not to attend group classes, then it would be wise to look under psychological implications of group therapy. Even if you cannot find any articles on the psychological implications of group exercise in osteoarthritis, you will be able to find articles on related subjects such as asthma, or low back pain; these may appear to be initially irrelevant but they may equally be valid since the science behind the articles will probably be talking about the psychology of chronic disease management. A later chapter explains how to search databases efficiently.

Have I used appropriate sources, and have I performed a critical analysis of the literature or is it a shopping list of the articles that I managed to get hold of?

- Do not list one piece of literature after another. Lecturers usually worry when they see every paragraph beginning with a string of references. For example:

  Smith (1999) found that childbirth was painful; Jones (2002) found that pain in childbirth was a problem; Johnson (2001) found that pain was significant in childbirth [etc.]

  Instead, organise the literature review into sections that present themes or identify any trends. You are not trying to list all the material published, but to synthesise it according to the overall concept of your research question. For example:

  Smith (1999), Jones (2002) and Johnson (2001) have all commented on pain levels following childbirth and their conclusions can be summarised as . . . moving onto the psychological aspects of childbirth, the main findings are. . . .

Have I cited and discussed studies whose findings may be contrary to my perspective?

- This is a useful thing to do since it provides balance to the work; you will probably never find complete agreement in the literature.

Can I highlight any gaps in the field?

- This is important, since it shows that you have a clear understanding of why your project is important. Having said that, ensure that you do not aim too high; you have limited time to undertake an undergraduate project.

ENDING YOUR
LITERATURE REVIEW

Many students end their literature reviews on a whimper, this is a shame, you should always try to summarise major contributions of significant studies under review, maintaining the focus that you set out right at the beginning, and evaluate the 'state of the art' for the subject pointing out any methodological flaws or gaps in research and areas or issues pertinent to future study. After all, if you have decided that further work needs to be done, this is your chance to argue your case.

SYNTHESISING THE LITERATURE INTO
YOUR OWN WORK

Students often struggle with how to synthesise literature. There is something of a paradox here – as an undergraduate you will probably not have done any research at all, let alone be in a position to comment on the work of others, yet you are expected to some degree to criticise, compliment or otherwise comment on the work of others. This is one of the reasons that you need to have a basic understanding of the research process. You must be able to recognise good research. Students often do not know what we mean by synthesis and this is an important cause of student failure, so before we go on further let us consider the example below.

Example: You are given a set of ingredients that could result in a fruitcake. You have two choices: you can either describe each ingredient, i.e. say what you

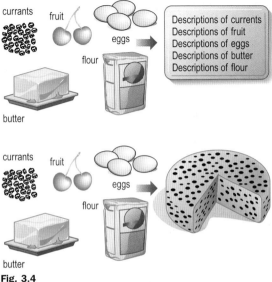

Fig. 3.4

see, or you can attempt to combine them into a mixture that sticks together – and while the original ingredients are still there, they have been combined and changed to something new (Fig. 3.4).

Now, to our research problem example: the use of group exercise in osteoarthritis of the knee. In place of ingredients, we can place our research articles. The diagram would now look something like this:

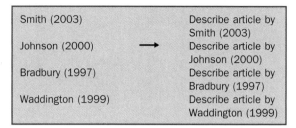

Again the result here is like the unmixed fruitcake, there is little meaning to the final work and the reader would be left with no clear idea about the state of group exercise in osteoarthritis. This type of literature review tends to read as nothing more than a list of articles.

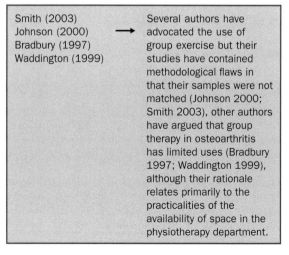

What happens if there is no literature to review?

Students sometimes say that they have performed a litera- ture search and there is no relevant literature to discuss – there are several answers to this problem:

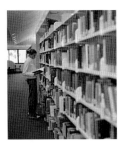

Fig. 3.5

1. You have not looked.
2. You have looked but in the wrong place.
3. You have looked in the right place but for the wrong specific information.
4. There really is no other literature on the subject?

Table 3.2 suggests some solutions.

READING ARTICLES

The first time you read an academic article can be daunt- ing. Students often state that they were bored or con- fused by what they had read; indeed there is no escaping the fact that research articles can appear dull and unin- teresting, but like most things, each article is written for a specific purpose and with a specific audience in mind, who will not find it boring. The problem that you have as a student, is that you are often forced into reading something that you would not normally want to read – and you are expected to comment on it. Students often do not know what to look for when reading an article, so I will present you with a checklist that you can use as a template, it is not perfect, and cannot be used for everything that you will read, but it is a useful skeleton.

TABLE 3.2 SOME SUGGESTED SOLUTIONS TO FIND LITERATURE FOR YOUR REVIEW

Problem	Solution
You do not know how to undertake a literature review	Go to your university library or study skills unit immediately and book yourself into a session on how to do a literature search
You do know how to do a literature review but you have searched in an incorrect fashion	Discuss with your supervisor and read the chapter in this book on searching databases effectively
Your search was too narrow	Expand it
You searched for irrelevant topics	Make sure that you are clear about your research project, your aims and objectives, and what you wish to explore – narrow it down
Wrong database has been used	Familiarise yourself with the search engines that are most useful for your topic, e.g. Psychinfo, MEDLINE, CINAHL and PEDro
Your chosen topic is so unusual that there actually is no available literature, e.g. there are no data on the psychological effects of time travel	Be careful, there will probably be a very good reason why it has never been done before; the project may be impractical, impossible, too costly, irrelevant, etc.

THE 'HOW-TO' GUIDE FOR CRITICAL APPRAISAL OF LITERATURE

■ Does the title give a clear guide for what is to follow? The title should be concise and precise

■ What is the theme or the broad aims of the piece of work in front of you?

■ Have the writers explained or justified why they have done this study?

■ Have they explained and summarised the previous literature in the subject area? (Did they set the scene?)

■ What is the research question? (only if appropriate, do not forget that there may not be a single clear question in certain types of research)

■ What is the study design? Is it qualitative, quantitative; is it a case study, a systematic review or some other format. More importantly, does the design fit the question?

■ Have the researchers used the right tool for the right job? Have they acknowledged any other methodological approaches that could have been taken? Have they acknowledged any limitations of the study?

■ How did the researchers collect their data? Did they perform a pilot study?

■ Have they discussed validity and reliability?

■ What was their sample size? Do they note inclusion and exclusion criteria if relevant?

■ How was sampling achieved and is the sample described thoroughly?

Continued

- Were there any ethical issues? Did they obtain consent?
- Are the statistical tests appropriate and are any graphs clearly presented?
- Has any level of statistical significance been used? What are the findings of the paper?
- Did they answer their own research question?
- Does it add to the body of existing knowledge?
- How has the author(s) interpreted their results?
- Have they made unsupported claims or missed important points?
- The 'so what' question. Was it worthwhile? Will it change anything about your work? Could it be used in your own future clinical practice?
- How can you integrate the article into your work?

WHEN LITERATURE REVIEWS GO WRONG

Take a look at the common errors that students make when constructing a literature review. We will use the example of back pain but any other clinical topic could be used equally well.

Remember the ideal funnel shape of your review.

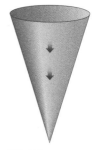

Fig. 3.6

Subject: Pain

This student wants to look at pain in general. This topic is too broad (see Fig. 3.7).

Consequence

This student runs the risk of going off at a tangent and giving the examiner plenty of ammunition for failure.

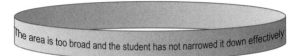

The area is too broad and the student has not narrowed it down effectively

Fig. 3.7

Subject: Back pain

Here (Fig. 3.8) the student wants to look at back pain but their literature review begins by discussing the prevalence of back pain in pregnancy, then goes on to the legal implications of back pain and then ends with a discussion on the structure of the spinal cord. Notice how these topics fall outside of the shaded area, in other words they are not relevant to the study, as a consequence

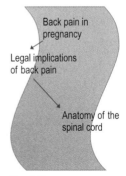

Back pain in pregnancy

Legal implications of back pain

Anatomy of the spinal cord

Fig. 3.8

there is no structure to the work, it is difficult to read and has no logical flow. It ends with a whimper, leaving the reader with no clear idea about the direction of the project. Also note that the funnel shape is absent, there is no point or direction to the literature review.

Consequence

This type of literature review makes the examiner feel uneasy as he or she does not know what is coming next. This student will be penalised for producing a piece of work that is unstructured with no clear research aim or question and no scene setting – in simpler terms you have not told a very good story.

Subject: Not clear

In this example (Fig. 3.9), the student has completed a good literature review on back pain, but has then chosen to do a project on arthritis of the neck. This sometimes happens when the student is unable to find suitable literature on their chosen topic – or is just being lazy.

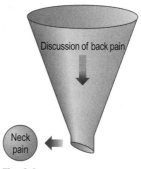

Fig. 3.9

Consequence

This student will lose marks for not having followed a clear path in their own research problem, rather like the previous example. They are likely to be perceived as having been lazy in not collecting the right type of literature, or worse still there is always the thought in the mind of the examiner that the work has been plagiarised from another source. Plagiarism is where somebody either deliberately or accidentally takes the work of someone else and passes it off as their own – universities take a very dim view of this.

HOW TO REFERENCE CORRECTLY

Poor referencing gives examiners headaches every year, so we are going to spend some time on how to avoid giving your examiner a headache!

What is a reference?

In the course of your studies you will be expected to acknowledge books, journal articles, etc. used in preparation for assignments, projects, essays and dissertations, by producing a list of references or a bibliography for each one. There are different conventions and as usual, you must make sure that you follow your college or university's guidelines as to which system they expect you to use, but the most common system is known as the Harvard system of referencing.

British Standards BS1629:1976 and BS5605:1990 define a bibliographical reference as:

'a set of data or elements describing a document, or part of a document, and sufficiently precise and detailed to enable a potential reader to identify and locate it'

Citing

Acknowledging within your text the document from which you have obtained your information.

Reference

The detailed description of the document from which you have obtained your information.

Why reference?

When writing reports or essays, you are expected to read around your subject. Referencing is a way of demonstrating that you have done that reading, that you know where it came from and that you acknowledge the authors as the creators of the work. Each time you use someone else's ideas or words, it is essential that you acknowledge this in your work. Not acknowledging other people's work is not only intellectually dishonest but also illegal. *Plagiarism* is the act of presenting the ideas or discoveries of another as one's own.

You should provide references:

- To acknowledge your sources
- To substantiate your arguments
- To avoid plagiarism, even when unintentional
- To enable your reader to follow-up your source material.

When to reference?

With thanks to Matt Holland and Bournemouth University Library for permission to use their Citing References Guide.

Whenever you use any source of information for:

- Inspiration
- Facts, theories, findings or ideas in another author's work

- Specific data or statistics
- Direct quotations
- Paraphrasing another author's words.

The following notes are based on British Standards: BS5605:1990. Recommendations for citing and referencing published material, 2nd ed. BSI (Talbot Campus Library & Learning Centre – 028.7 BRI) BS1629:1989. Recommendations for references to published materials. BSI (Bournemouth House Library and Talbot Campus Library & Learning Centre – 028.7 BRI).

When writing a piece of work, you will need to refer in your text to material written or produced by others. This procedure is called citing or quoting references. Consistency and accuracy are important to enable readers to identify and locate the material to which you have referred. The same set of rules should be followed every time you cite a reference.

THE HARVARD SYSTEM OF REFERENCING

All statements, opinions, conclusions, etc. taken from another writer's work should be cited, whether the work is directly quoted, paraphrased or summarised. In the Harvard system, cited publications are referred to in the text by giving the author's surname and the year of publication and are listed in a bibliography at the end of the text.

Originators/authors: the person or organisation shown most prominently in the source as responsible for the content in its published form should be given. For anonymous works, use 'Anon' instead of a name. For certain kinds of work, e.g. dictionaries or encyclopaedias, or if an item is the cooperative work of many individuals, none of whom have a dominant role, e.g. videos or films, the title may be used instead of an originator or author.

Dates: if an exact year or date is not known, an approximate date preceded by 'ca.' may be supplied and given in square brackets. If no such approximation is possible, that should be stated, e.g. [ca. 1750] or [no date].

All examples within this chapter are fictitious and any resemblance to existing works is coincidental.

References in the text
Quotations
As a general rule in the university, if the quote is less than a line, it may be included in the body of the text in quotation marks. Longer quotations are indented and single-spaced, quotation marks are not required. For citations of particular parts of the document, the page numbers etc. should be given in parentheses, after the year.

Summaries or paraphrases
Give the citation where it occurs naturally, or at the end of the relevant piece of writing. Diagrams and illustrations should be referenced as though they were a quotation if they have been taken from a published work. For anything else, refer to BS1629:1989.

If an electronic document does not include pagination or an equivalent internal referencing system, the extent of the item may be indicated in terms such as the total number of lines, screens, etc., e.g. '[35 lines]' or '[approx. 12 screens]'.

Examples

1. If the author's name occurs naturally in the
    sentence, the year is given in parentheses,
    e.g. In a popular study, Harvey (1992) argued
      that we have to teach good practices . . .;
    e.g. As Harvey (1992, p. 21) said, 'good practices
      must be taught' and so we . . .

2. If the name does not occur naturally in the
    sentence, both name and year are given in
    parentheses:
    e.g. A more recent study (Stevens 1998) has
      shown the way theory and practical work
      interact.
    e.g. Theory rises out of practice, and once
      validated, returns to direct or explain the
      practice (Stevens 1998).

3. When an author has published more than one
    cited document in the same year, these are
    distinguished by adding lower case letters (a, b,
    c, etc.) after the year and within the parentheses:
    e.g. Johnson (1994a) discussed the subject . . .

4. If there are two authors, the surnames of both
    should be given:
    e.g. Matthews and Jones (1997) have proposed
      that . . .

5. If there are more than two authors, the surname
    of the first author only should be given, followed
    by et al.:
    e.g. Office costs amount to 20% of total costs in
      most businesses (Wilson et al. 1997)

(You should complete a full listing of names in the bibliography at the end.)

6. If the work is anonymous, then 'Anon' should be used:

   e.g. In a recent article (Anon 1998) it was stated that . . .

7. If it is a reference to a newspaper article with no author, the name of the paper can be used in place of 'Anon':

   e.g. More people than ever seem to be using retail home delivery (*The Times* 1996)

   (You should use the same style in the bibliography.)

8. If you refer to a source quoted in another source, you cite both in the text:

   e.g. A study by Smith (1960, cited in Jones 1994) showed that . . .

   (You should list only the work you have read, i.e. Jones, in the bibliography.)

9. If you refer to a contributor in a source, you cite just the contributor:

   e.g. Software development has been given as the cornerstone in this industry (Bantz 1995).

10. If you refer to a person who has not produced a work, or contributed to one, but who is quoted in someone else's work it is suggested that you should mention the person's name and you must cite the source author:

    e.g. Richard Hammond stressed the part psychology plays in advertising in an interview with Marshall (1999).

e.g. 'Advertising will always play on peoples'
    desires', Richard Hammond said in a recent
    article (Marshall 1999, p. 67).
(You should list the work that has been
    published, i.e. Marshall, in the bibliography.)

Personal communications

*Adapted from: APA 1983. Publication Manual of the
American Psychological Association. 3rd ed. Washington:
APA.*

They do not provide recoverable data and so are not
included in the reference list. Cite personal communications in the text only. Give initials as well as the surname
of the communicator and provide as exact a date as
possible.

e.g. Many patients do not do their exercises according to S. Porter (personal communication, 19 April,
2006) [pers. comm. is sometimes used].

References at the end of a piece of work

At the end of a piece of work, list references to documents cited in the text. This list may be called a Bibliography or more commonly, References. Exceptionally
you may be asked to list references not cited in the text
but which make an important contribution to your
work. These are usually listed under the heading of
Further Reading. You are advised to review the guidelines issued to you for the preparation of work to clarify
this point.

In the Harvard system, the references are listed in
alphabetical order of authors' names. If you have cited
more than one item by a specific author they should
be listed chronologically (earliest first), and by letter

(1993a, 1993b) if more than one item has been published during a specific year.

Whenever possible, elements of a bibliographical reference should be taken from the title page of the publication.

For place of publication give the city. If more than one town/city is listed, give the first one or the location of the publisher's head office. If the town/city is not well known, you may in addition add a county, region or state. Note that in the USA, states are denoted by a two letter code, for example Hillsdale, NJ. For the publisher's name, omit superfluous terms such as Publishers, Co, or Inc. Always retain the words Books or Press. Where the publisher is a university and the place or location is included in the name of the university, do not repeat the place of publication.

Each reference should use the elements and punctuation given in the following examples for the different types of published work you may have cited. Underlining is an acceptable alternative to italics when bibliographies are hand written.

Reference to a book
Author's SURNAME, INITIALS, Year of publication. Title. Edition (if not the first). Place of publication: Publisher.
e.g. Mercer, P.A. and Smith, G. 1993. Private viewdata in the UK. 2nd ed. London: Longman.

Reference to a contribution in a book
Contributing author's SURNAME, INITIALS, Year of publication. Title of contribution. Followed by In: INITIALS, SURNAME of author or editor of publication

followed by ed. or eds if relevant. Title of book. Place of publication: Publisher, Page number(s) of contribution.

e.g. BANTZ, C.R. 1995. Social dimensions of software development. In: J.A. ANDERSON, ed. Annual review of software management and development. Newbury Park, CA: SAGE, 502–510.

Reference to an article in a journal

Author's SURNAME, INITIALS, Year of publication. Title of article. Title of Journal, Volume number and (part number), page numbers of contribution.

e.g. EVANS, W.A. 1994. Approaches to intelligent information retrieval. Information Processing and Management 7(2), 147–168.

Reference to a newspaper article

Author's SURNAME, INITIALS (or NEWSPAPER TITLE), Year of publication. Title of article. Title of newspaper, Day and month, Page number/s and column number.

e.g. INDEPENDENT 1992. Picking up the bills. Independent, 4 June, p. 28a.

Reference to a conference paper

Contributing author's SURNAME, INITIALS, Year of publication. Title of contribution. Followed by In: INITIALS, SURNAME of editor of proceedings (if applicable) followed by ed. Title of conference proceedings including date and place of conference. Place of publication: Publisher, page numbers of contribution.

e.g. SILVER, K. 1991. Electronic mail: the new way to communicate. In: D.I. RAITT, ed. 9th international online information meeting, 3–5 December 1990. London. Oxford: Learned Information 323–330.

Reference to a publication from a corporate body (e.g. a government department or other organisation)

NAME OF ISSUING BODY, Year of publication. Title of publication. Place of publication: Publisher, Report Number (where relevant).

e.g. UNESCO 1993. General information programme and UNISIST. Paris: UNESCO (PGI-93/WS/22).

Reference to a thesis

Author's SURNAME, INITIALS, Year of publication. Title of thesis. Designation (and type). Name of institution to which submitted.

e.g. AGUTTER, A.J. 1995. The linguistic significance of current British slang. Thesis (PhD). Edinburgh University.

Reference to a patent

ORIGINATOR (name of applicant). Year of publication. Title of patent. Series designation, which may include full date.

e.g. PHILIP MORRIS INC. 1981. Optical perforating apparatus and system. European patent application 0021165 A1. 1981-01-07.

Reference to a video, film or broadcast

Title, Year. (For films, the preferred date is the year of release in the country of production.) Material designation. Subsidiary originator. (Optional but director is preferred, SURNAME in capitals). Production details – place: organisation.

e.g. Macbeth, 1948. Film. Directed by Orson Welles. USA: Republic Pictures.

e.g. Birds in the Garden, 1998. Video. London: Harper Videos.

Programmes and series: the number and title of the episode should normally be given, as well as the series title, the transmitting organisation and channel, the full date and time of transmission.

e.g. Yes, Prime Minister, Episode 1, The Ministerial Broadcast, 1986. TV, BBC2. 1986 16 Jan.

e.g. News at Ten, 2001. 27 Jan, 2200 hrs.

Contributions: individual items within a programme should be cited as contributors.

e.g. BLAIR, Tony, 1997. Interview. In: Six O'clock News. TV, BBC1. 1997 29 Feb. 1823 hrs.

Electronic material – following the Harvard system

The British Standard BS 5605:1990 does not include recommendations for electronic sources. The recommendations in this document follow best practice in referencing electronic resources and where possible follow the guidance of the British Standard.

Reference to web pages/sites and e-books

Author's /editor's SURNAME, INITIALS, Year. Title [online]. (Edition). Place of publication, Publisher (if ascertainable). Available from: URL [Accessed date].

e.g. HOLLAND, M, 2004. Guide to citing Internet sources [online]. Poole, Bournemouth University. Available from: http://www.bournemouth.ac.uk/ library/using/guide_to_citing_internet_sourc.html [Accessed 4 November 2004].

Reference to e-journals

Author's SURNAME, INITIALS, Year. Title. Journal Title [online], volume (issue), location within host. Available from: URL [Accessed date].

e.g. KORB, K.B. 1995. Persons and things: book review of Bringsjord on Robot-Consciousness. Psycoloquy [online], 6 (15). Available from: http://psycprints.ecs.soton.ac.uk/archive/ 00000462/ [Accessed 20 May 2004].

Reference to mailbase/listserv e-mail lists

Author's SURNAME, INITIALS, Day Month Year. Subject of message. Discussion List [online]. Available from: list e-mail address [Accessed date].

e.g. BRACK, E.V. 2 May 2004. Re: Computing short courses. Lis-link [online]. Available from: jiscmail@jiscmail.ac.uk [Accessed 17 Jun 2004].

e.g. JENSEN, L.R. 12 Dec 1999. Recommendation of student radio/tv in English. IASTAR [online]. Available from: LISTSERV@FTP.NRG.DTU.DK [Accessed 29 Apr 2004].

It should be noted that items may only be kept on discussion group servers for a short time and hence may not be suitable for referencing. A local copy could be kept by the author who is giving the citation, with a note to this effect.

Reference to personal electronic communications (e-mail)

Sender's SURNAME, INITIALS (Sender's e-mail address), Day Month Year. Subject of Message. e-mail to recipient's INITIALS. SURNAME (Recipient's e-mail address).

e.g. LOWMAN, D. (deborah_lowman@pbsinc.com),
    4 Apr 2000. RE: ProCite and Internet Reference.
    e-Mail to P. CROSS (pcross@bournemouth.ac.uk).

Reference to CD-ROMs and DVDs

This section refers to CD-ROMs which are works in their own right and not bibliographic databases.

Author's SURNAME, INITIALS, Year. Title [type of medium CD-ROM]. (Edition). Place of publication, Publisher (if ascertainable). Available from: Supplier/Database identifier or number (optional) [Accessed Date] (optional).

e.g. HAWKING, S.W. 1994. A brief history of time:
    an interactive adventure. [CD-ROM]. Crunch
    Media.

Citing unpublished material

See BS6371:1983. Citation of unpublished documents. BSI (Talbot Campus Library & Learning Centre and Bournemouth House Library 028.7 BRI).

PLAGIARISM

Remember that you must acknowledge your source every time you refer to someone else's work. Failure to do so amounts to plagiarism, which is against the university rules and is a serious offence.

ESSAY WRITING

Sally French and John Swain

Northedge defines an essay as '. . . a short piece of writing on a specific subject' (1996:110). You are frequently required to write essays as a means of demonstrating your mastery of a particular topic and your ability to express ideas coherently and in your own words. It is often the means by which you are assessed. Writing is demanding as it involves the development, shaping and expression of our thoughts and understandings. It is an active, dynamic process which takes considerable time, practice, patience and effort to perfect.

Constructing an essay does, however, demand skills other than the ability to write. It usually starts with note taking where relevant material for the essay is gathered. At this stage, it is crucial to read and select material that enables you to respond to the title precisely. A common mistake in essay writing is to pay insufficient attention to what is being asked. It is advisable, therefore, to highlight keywords in the title to avoid the possibility of 'going off on a tangent'. The words you underline should be 'content' words (which indicate what you must write about) and 'command' or 'process' words (which indicate what you should do with the content you select). In the following examples, the content words are underlined and the command words are in italics:

Evaluate the use of <u>mobilisations</u> in the <u>treatment</u> of <u>capsulitis</u> of the <u>shoulder</u>.

Justify the use of <u>behaviour modification</u> in the <u>treatment</u> of patients following <u>brain injury</u>.

The command word *evaluate* is asking you to appraise the effectiveness or worth of mobilisations in the treatment of capsulitis of the shoulder. The content words are directing you to a particular medical condition (capsulitis), which is affecting a specific part of the body (the shoulder). You are not, therefore, being asked to consider capsulitis in any other joint or any other condition that might effect the shoulder. The command word *justify* in the second example, is asking you to provide grounds for the use of behaviour modification and to raise and allay any objections to it. The content words are directing you to a particular intervention (behaviour modification) in a particular circumstance (following brain injury). You are not being asked to consider behaviour modification for other patient groups or other interventions for people with brain injury.

Essay titles such as these also contain, implicitly, a controversy for you to consider. The first essay title implies that there are arguments both for and against the use of mobilisations in the treatment of capsulitis of the shoulder with the likelihood of research articles supporting both opinions. The second essay title implies that there are objections to the use of behaviour modification following brain injury, on ethical grounds perhaps, as well as arguments that support it. Rather than coming down strongly on one side or the other, you are being asked to consider the evidence and to show that you have 'read round' the subject and understood it. It is always advisable to read carefully any guidance notes you are given on how to tackle the essay and what is expected of you. As you read around, keep careful notes about the literature and other sources you consult. It can be frustrating to have noted a quotation without the full information to reference the source (especially when you have returned the book to the library).

Before you start reading and selecting appropriate material, it can be helpful to jot down all the ideas you have on the subject which you have accumulated from formal teaching, clinical education and your own experience. This will help you to get started and reassure you that you know something about the subject. Although it is likely that you will discard some of your jottings, other ideas and concepts will be important. You may organise them into 'mindmaps', where the central idea is placed in the middle of the page with branches and arrows radiating outwards showing how the ideas and concepts are connected. This is an alternative to linear notes and may be more representative of our thought patterns in the early stages of formulating ideas.

It is very important when writing essays to express the ideas in your own words. The ability to do this depends on your note-taking skills and how well you understand the ideas. As Poole and Kelly state '. . . in order to develop the skill of writing in your own words you need to read actively processing meaning as you go' (2004:43). Using somebody else's words and passing them off as your own is known as plagiarism. Although this is often done innocently, and usually indicates a weakness in note-taking skills and understanding, it can also be regarded as a form of cheating and must always be avoided as severe penalties can ensue. In order to avoid plagiarism, quotation marks must be placed around direct quotations and an indication made in the text of where important ideas have originated. This is usually done by placing the author's or researcher's name and date of their work in brackets. It is not acceptable to change the odd word or phase in somebody else's writing, as this is still regarded as plagiarism. Most institutions have strict rules often in course handbooks and it is important to familiarise yourself with these.

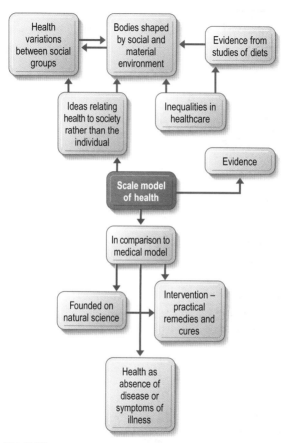

Fig. 3.10

As we have already discussed, your essay should demonstrate that you have grasped important ideas, that you have analysed the evidence and that you have constructed a coherent argument. It will usually be necessary to draw upon material that you have covered in your course. It can be powerful to use examples from your own experience but if this is done, it is important to relate it to the theories or evidence that you are considering. You may, for example, recall a patient you treated with mobilisations for capsulitis of the shoulder and discuss the outcome of your treatment with reference to the research evidence. Similarly, you may have worked in a unit for people with brain injury where behaviour modification was used and relate this to various ethical considerations or to a particular theoretical perspective. Sweeping statements, based on your own opinions or experience, should generally be avoided.

A common question from students is, 'should I put in my own opinions?' What really matters is the quality of the argument, not what you personally believe one way or the other. For instance, if you personally take the position that there will always be a place for special schools in educational provision, it is your basis for your views (literature, argument, evidence, views of others, etc.) and also how you deal with counter-arguments that counts.

As we discussed above, it is important that your essay is your own work and not copied from the work of fellow students or published authors. It is wrong, however, to consider writing as necessarily a solitary activity. If you are experiencing problems in writing, or wish to improve your marks, support of various kinds can be helpful. This will depend both on the institution where you are studying and your own particular circumstances. The first source of support can be your tutor. If your tutor offers support in this way, it can be useful to ask for a tutorial and to take along a plan of your essay and an introduction. Some students experience difficulties in expressing ideas in writing to such an extent that poor grammar, spelling and punctuation can be a barrier to the marker in understanding what the student is trying to say. This can be the case for people writing in a second language and for those who have dyslexia for instance. Some universities and colleges offer specific support services that can be called upon. In general, you can seek out and use different sources of support, while retaining the key principle that this is your piece of work, your ideas, in your own words.

You may also experience difficulties with time-management. This is especially true when the workload is high and a number of assignments need handing in around the same time. Time management is the key to ensuring that you organise your work to allow sufficient time for each of your writing tasks. A calendar can help in setting yourself personal deadlines for each aspect of your work.

Structuring essays

It is important that your essay is structured so that your ideas flow and the people reading it (who are frequently assessing your work) can understand what you are saying. It is wise to plan your essay before you write it, although the plan may change and develop once you start. Most essays are structured in the following way:

- Title
- Introduction
- Main section
- Conclusion
- References.

However, Redman states that:

. . . an essay is always greater than its component parts, and it is how you put all those parts together that is often as important as the parts themselves (2001:18)

We have assumed that the title of the essay will be given to you but you may, on occasions, be required to create a title of your own. In such circumstances, it can help to check out your title with your tutor. As mentioned already, it is vitally important that you respond to the title of the essay precisely to whoever has constructed it. It is good practice always to include the full, exact title at the top of your essay. Some set titles provide a quotation followed by a process word, such as 'discuss'. You should give the full quotation including, where possible, the reference for the source of the quotation.

The introduction is more important than is generally recognised. It is not unusual to mark essays without an introduction or with a minimal couple of sentences to set the scene. For instance, we have marked essays that begin with a summary of the history of a topic with no explanation of where the discussion is going or why such a history is relevant to the particular issues being addressed. In the introduction you should show that you understand what is expected of you and briefly explain what you intend to do and how you are going to do it. Going back to the first of our two essay titles, you may indicate your understanding that there is a debate around the use of mobilisations in the treatment of capsulitis of the shoulder and that you are going to analyse the evidence from both sides. It may also be necessary to define key terms in the introduction, especially those that are contested. If you were writing an essay about disability, for example, it may be necessary to define the meaning of the word as it means different things to different people.

As the introduction should clearly state what you intend to do in the essay, it can be difficult to write it first (when the exact content of your essay is unclear). Redman points out that this is in no way necessary:

The difficulty with introduction writing is that sometimes you only know what the core arguments are when you have finished your essay. So, although writing the introduction can help to give you a clear idea of what you are doing, you may find it is a good idea to write it last. (2001:46)

As you progress through your course, you may be encouraged to argue an issue from a particular position of your choice rather than presenting both sides of an argument. If this is the case, you need to indicate in the introduction the line you intend to take. If, for example, you were presented with the following essay title: 'Physiotherapists play an important role in the ability of disabled people to become and remain independent. Discuss this claim with reference to one model of disability', you may decide to argue from the perspective of the social model rather than the medical model of disability. You can also state a particular focus for your essay. For instance, given this title, you may wish to focus on people with learning difficulties. This can strengthen your essay if the focus is clearly defined in your introduction and you can justify it. You might argue that the issues have particular pertinence to physiotherapists working with people with learning difficulties or that you have personal experience of work in this area.

When the title includes a quotation, it is useful to consult and refer to the original source. It may be, for instance, that the quotation is from a paper based on research undertaken by the author(s). In this case, a sentence or two outlining the nature of the research can help put the quotation in context and set the scene for your discussion.

The main section of your essay is the longest part and is where you present the bulk of your material. It is here where you construct your argument, being sure to engage with the title of the essay at all times and examining the issue from different points of view and theoretical perspectives. You will need to present and evaluate evidence and theory and may make use of your own experience if this is appropriate. You need to select the most important material to support your argument, which may include maps, numerical data and diagrams. As you will have a specific word count, your ability to précis material and write succinctly will be tested to the full.

The conclusion of your essay is usually no more than a paragraph or two in length. It is here that you need to summarise the main content of your essay and recap the core arguments. A good tactic in writing your conclusion is to return to your introduction and the title of the essay. This pulls the whole analysis and argument together, and makes it clear that you have directly addressed the specific title. It is important not to raise new issues in your conclusion, i.e. issues that have not been discussed in the body of the essay. You may, however, point out areas in the debate that need developing.

At the end of your essay you should list in full the references that you have used and which appear in the text. There are various styles in which references are presented, the most common one being the Harvard system. The important thing is that all the information is present so that interested readers can look up the references if they wish. Some university and college libraries have booklets for students outlining the 'house style' for referencing for the institution. A list of references also indicates that you have engaged with the literature. The references you cite should always be relevant to what you are discussing and should generally be up-to-date. (For a full discussion of referencing styles, see French and Sim 1993 and Northedge 1996).

Making your essay flow

As well as attending to content, your essay should also be fluent and easy to read. This can be achieved in many ways, some of which have already been discussed. Outlining what you intend to do in the introduction, defining key terms, and structuring your essay logically will all help the reader to follow your line of argument. Clear explanations and providing examples to illustrate the points you are making will help to give clarity and focus. Short sentences and simple language are also important in getting your meaning across. As Redman states:

There is nothing to be gained from using complex language for its own sake. The real test lies in being able to communicate complex ideas in the form that is most easily understood. (2001:65–66)

Jargon and the excessive use of abbreviations should be avoided and paragraphs should be kept short and should generally contain just one major theme. Varying the length of sentences and paragraphs does, however, give your writing rhythm. The use of sub-headings can also help to structure your argument.

Keeping your readers on track is sometimes referred to as 'signposting'. You constantly need to discreetly remind your readers of what you are doing, so that they do not lose the thread of your argument. A sound introduction and overall structure will assist with this but you can also use 'linking' words and phrases to help your essay flow. Phrases such as 'as we have seen', 'on the other hand', 'to summarise', 'to conclude' and 'before we discuss x we need to consider y', all inform your readers of where you are going. Linking words such as 'therefore', 'nevertheless', 'conversely', 'however' also serve the purpose of linking together the ideas you are presenting. It is a good strategy to imagine that you are writing for the 'intelligent lay person' rather than your tutor. In that way, points that may seem too obvious to mention will not be omitted. The overall presentation of your essay is also important. Handwriting should be clear, font size comfortable to read, and margins wide enough to allow for the writing of comments. The correct level of formality or informality of your essay, e.g. whether you write in the first person, varies across academic disciplines. Generally, the 'hard' sciences, such as physiology and physics, take a more formal stance than the social sciences.

It will usually be necessary to write at least two drafts before handing your essay in. In the first draft, you need to concentrate on the content and overall structure of your essay and in the second draft, you need to think about your reader and attend to the clarity of your writing, including your spelling and punctuation. Considerable cutting and rearranging usually takes place at this stage. Both content and style are important in achieving a good grade.

CONCLUSION

As we mentioned at the beginning of this chapter, the skill of writing well is not easy and takes considerable time and effort. The rewards of writing are, however, great. Because you have engaged in a dynamic and challenging activity, your understanding of the topic, as well as your memory of the issues, will be enhanced. Furthermore, you will have practised a skill which is so important in the work of physiotherapists today.

LEARNING OUTCOMES

After reading this chapter you should have a basic understanding of . . .

- What a literature review is
- How to back up your arguments
- The qualities of a good literature review
- Questions to ask yourself
- How to end your literature review
- How to synthesise the available literature

- How to read and appraise literature
- When literature reviews go wrong – what to avoid
- How to reference – guidance on the Harvard system
- How to write essays.

REFERENCES

French S, Sim J 1993 Writing: a guide for therapists. Butterworth-Heinemann, Oxford.

Northedge A 1996 The good study guide. Open University, Milton Keynes.

Poole L, Kelly B 2004 Preparing to study DD100/DD121. Reading and note taking. Open University, Milton Keynes.

Redman P 2001 Good essay writing: a social science guide. SAGE, London.

How to search databases

Mark Elkins

If physicians would read two articles per day out of the six million medical articles published annually, in one year, they would fall 82 centuries behind in their reading.

(Miser 1999)

The amount of health-related research that is published is enormous and expanding exponentially. This is true even of the physiotherapy literature alone (Herbert et al. 2001; Moseley et al. 2002).

You will never keep up if you try to read everything. You could easily use up the time you have available for reading research just scanning journals to see what has been published. You need to use your time more efficiently. This chapter will describe some strategies to help you maximise the amount of useful information you can obtain during the time you have available to read research.

DECIDING WHAT TO READ

There are several reasons you might be interested in reading published research, e.g.:

- You have been given an assignment on a particular disorder or treatment
- You have a patient and would like to know which treatments have been proven helpful for their condition
- You are planning some research of your own and want to know whether the trial you have in mind has already been performed.

Each of these circumstances affects the type of publications you will want to read. If you are new to the topic in question, it would be wise to start with some background information. Textbooks often provide comprehensive introductions to a disease: what causes it, how common it is, how it is diagnosed, and what effects it has on the patient. Similarly, if you are unfamiliar with a particular treatment, textbooks often provide detailed descriptions of how the treatment should be applied, what outcome it is designed to influence, and so on. Any library linked to a university or hospital will provide a catalogue and referencing system that will help you track down an appropriate textbook. You are probably familiar with this process. If not, speak to your librarian or enrol in a class to familiarise yourself.

Many textbooks or other sources of high-quality, background information are also available on the internet. Unfortunately, there is plenty of disreputable and inaccurate information on the internet as well. Here is a checklist for deciding whether the content of a health-related website is likely to be accurate:

- The site should be maintained by a credible organisation, like a national medical society or association, a government agency, or a university health centre
- Authors should display their credentials
- A site that sells or advertises treatments, especially if the retailer has also provided the main content, may be open to bias
- The site should identify when the information was posted and how regularly the content is reviewed and, if necessary, updated.

Chat rooms and bulletin boards generally provide information based on personal experience. Even if some accurate information were discussed, you would need to go to the original source to confirm its authenticity. Often sites with high-quality, up-to-date information require a subscription, so investigate what internet-based resources are available through your institution.

If you are familiar with a disorder and how to apply various treatments, but seek the best evidence on how effective the treatments are, you are unlikely to find useful information in textbooks. Whether electronic or hardcopy, textbooks take a long time to compile, yet the body of research into possible treatments is expanding and changing rapidly. Thus, many textbooks that discuss management of disorders are often outdated by the time they are published. Journals publish more rapidly and are a better source of original, up-to-date material.

SEARCHING JOURNALS EFFICIENTLY

Some skill is required to find the material you want in journals. Because journals publish research as it becomes available, the articles in a single edition tend to be quite unrelated. Journals vary in how their content is defined. Some include any papers within a discipline (e.g. *Australian Journal of Physiotherapy*). Others restrict their content to a particular patient group, by age (e.g. *Pediatric Clinics of North America*), by disease (e.g. *Journal of Cystic Fibrosis*), by symptom (e.g. *Pain*), or by treatment (e.g. *Manual Therapy*). This variability causes a high degree of overlap of content areas among journals. If you wished to know, for example, whether manual therapy would reduce joint pains in a child with cystic fibrosis, relevant research papers might be found in any edition of these and many other relevant journals. Scanning editions by hand will not do. The rest of this chapter is divided into four sections that discuss ways to search efficiently for information.

EFFICIENCY TIP NO. 1: USE ELECTRONIC DATABASES TO SEARCH Several databases are available on the internet to assist you in searching for articles published in journals. These databases contain a standard set of details about each article in thousands of journals. Typically, these details include the title of the article, the authors' names, an abstract (a one paragraph summary of the content of the article), and the citation details (the journal name, the year of publication, the edition number, and the page number). In addition, each article may be given keywords – a list of terms that describe the general content area of the article, even though such words may not appear in the title or even in the abstract. Sometimes the authors choose keywords and publish them with the article. Alternatively, database compilers may apply their own. The keywords and the other details mentioned above are stored in fields: the author field contains the authors' names; the keyword field contains the keywords, and so on.

A database will allow you to enter words, called search terms, that you would expect to appear in one of the fields. If you imagine the type of article that would give you the information you want, a few words from the title would make suitable search terms. For example, if you would like to know whether exercise is beneficial for low back pain in pregnant women, you could try *low back pain* and *pregnancy* as your search terms.

SEARCHING MEDLINE EFFICIENTLY

The largest and best known database is MEDLINE. There are several versions of MEDLINE which all contain basically the same information – details of articles from a wide and comprehensive selection of biomedicine and allied health journals. The main differences among the versions of MEDLINE relate to the search interface – the appearance of the search screens and how they function.

Let us now look at how to enter search terms in one version of MEDLINE, called PubMed. The home page of PubMed is http://www.ncbi.nlm.nih.gov/entrez/ query.fcgi, from which you can perform a simple search. Just type your search terms into the box near the top of the screen and click 'Go', as shown in Figure 4.1.

The graphics in Figure 4.1 are displayed with kind permission from the US National Library of Medicine (NLM).

The database searches the fields of each article for the search terms. If all the search terms are found in an article, it is retrieved by the database. The authors, title and citation details of all the retrieved articles are then displayed on the screen, as shown in Figure 4.2.

The most recently published articles are listed first. If you scroll down the list, you can look for titles that suggest they contain the information you want. As you do this, you will notice great variety in the types of articles returned: epidemiological studies, case reports, surveys, clinical trials, reviews, letters to the editor, and so on. Since our example related to the efficacy of a treatment, in this case we are probably interested in clinical trials. As you browse the list, you may notice an article that looks promising. If you click on the list of authors, it will bring up a more complete record, which includes all the citation details, the abstract and, in this case, a link to the website of the publisher, as shown in Figure 4.3. This link will often lead you to an electronic version of the full text of the article.

If the article is of interest to you, you can click the small box on the left, which 'selects' the article. Selecting articles as you browse the list allows you to easily return to them later. If you find an article that is a particularly good example of the type of article you wish to find, you can click on 'Related Articles'. This will

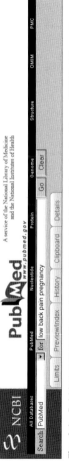

Fig. 4.1 PubMed web page: search box (Figs 4.1–4.7 with thanks to J Levy, CINAHL Information Systems, Glendale, California – MEDLINE).

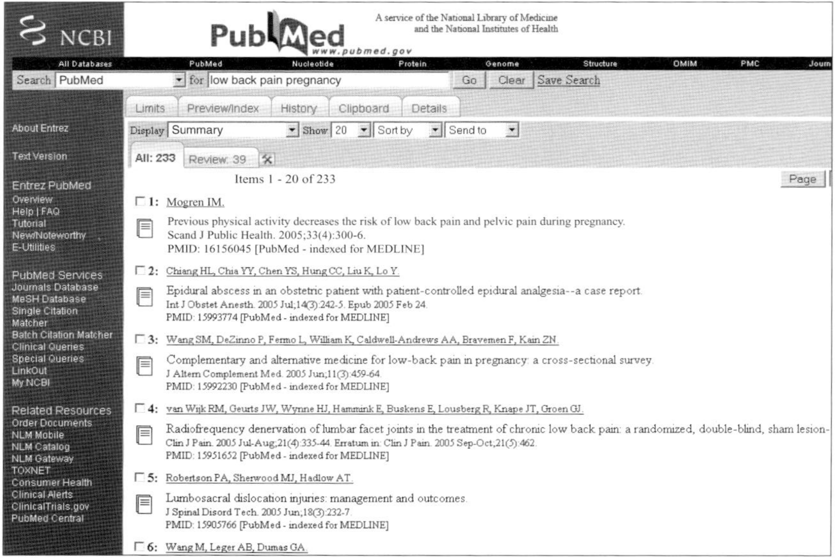

Fig. 4.2 PubMed web page: search results.

Related Articles, Links

☐ 1: Int J Gynaecol Obstet. 2005 Mar;88(3):271-5. Epub 2005 Jan 16.

ELSEVIER
FULL TEXT ARTICLE

The effect of exercise on the intensity of low back pain in pregnant women.

Garshasbi A, Faghih Zadeh S.

Department of Obstetrics and Gynecology, Shahed University, Faculty of Medicine, 1481973411 Tehran, Iran. agarshasbi@obgyn.net

OBJECTIVE: To investigate the effect of exercise during pregnancy on the intensity of low back pain and kinematics of spine. METHOD: A prospective randomized study was designed. 107 women participated in an exercise program three times a week during second half of pregnancy for 12 weeks and 105 as control group. All filled a questionnaire between 17-22 weeks of gestation and 12 weeks later for assessment of their back pain intensity. Lordosis and flexibility of spine were measured by Flexible ruler and Side bending test, respectively, at the same times. Weight gain during pregnancy, Pregnancy length and neonatal weight were recorded. RESULT: Low back pain intensity was increased in the control group. The exercise group showed significant reduction in the intensity of low back pain after exercise (p<0.0001). Flexibility of spine decreased more in the exercise group (p<0.0001). Weight gain during pregnancy, pregnancy length and neonatal weight were not different between the two groups. CONCLUSION: Exercise during second half of the pregnancy significantly reduced the intensity of low back pain, had no detectable effect on lordosis and had significant effect on flexibility of spine.

Fig. 4.3 PubMed web page: single article.

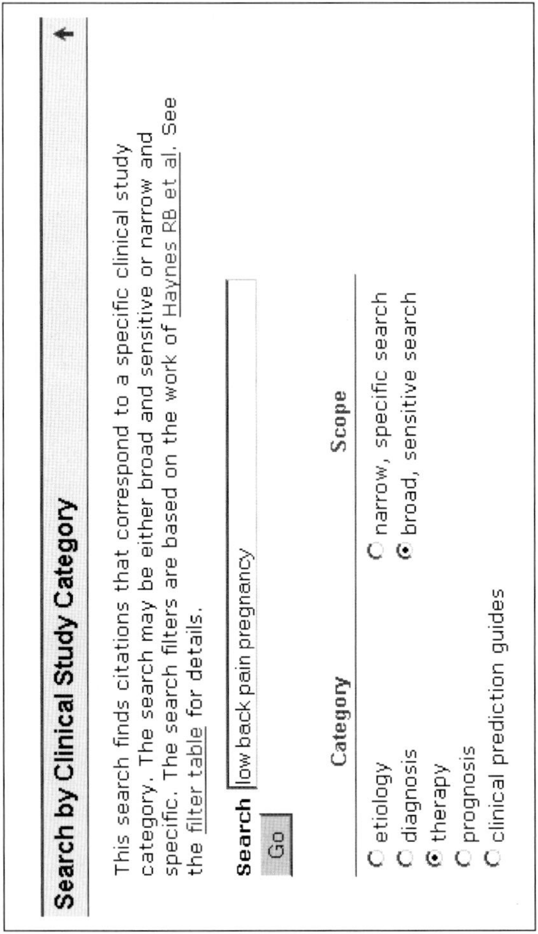

Fig. 4.4 PubMed web page: clinical study search for trials of therapies.

return a list of articles with the same keywords. For this example, this strategy retrieves several relevant trials.

There are other ways to refine your search. If you add *exercise* to the list of search terms then, not surprisingly, a greater proportion of the retrieved articles are relevant. There is still a mixture of study designs: case reports, surveys, prognostic studies, clinical studies, and so on. PubMed offers a simple way to refine this aspect of your search. In the left margin is a service called 'Clinical Queries'. This gives you the opportunity to restrict your search to a particular type of clinical study. If you select, e.g. 'therapy', you can restrict the retrieved articles to clinical trials of therapeutic interventions.

The scope of the search can be defined in the same place. If your search retrieves too great a proportion of irrelevant trials, try selecting the 'narrow, specific search' option. Alternatively, if a very small number of highly relevant trials are retrieved, try the 'broad, sensitive search' option. Ideally, your search will have a fairly high proportion of relevant articles, with a few less-relevant ones suggesting that you have captured all or most of the relevant trials, as shown in Figure 4.4.

EFFICIENCY TIP NO. 2: DEFINE THE QUESTION YOU WANT TO ANSWER WITH YOUR SEARCH   Reading journals is a bit like surfing the internet. Just as there are links from site to site, each article contains references which direct you to other related articles. Like internet links, the references can help you find the material you want or distract you from it. At the outset, decide on a question that it is most important for you to answer – it will help you to stay focussed. If you find interesting side issues as you search, you can note them and investigate them another time.

Another advantage of defining your question is that it identifies possible search terms. You should, however, also consider other terms that might be used to refer to the key concepts in your question. Suppose you were interested to know what proportion of people had returned to employment 1 year after surviving a stroke. If you use *employment* as a search term, you would miss an article that only used the word *employed*. This problem can be solved with 'wildcards' – symbols that can be attached to search terms and that allow any string of letters to take their place during the search.

SEARCHING CINAHL EFFICIENTLY

Let us look at another database, CINAHL, which offers wildcards. CINAHL, which stands for the Cumulative Index of Nursing and Allied Health Literature, indexes literature related to nursing, allied health, consumer health and biomedicine.

One wildcard offered by CINAHL is the '$' sign – which truncates the word. Thus *employ$* would retrieve both *employed* and *employment*. Different databases offer wildcards that operate slightly differently. Some use the '@' sign to represent a single character, so *randomi@ed* would retrieve *randomised* and *randomized*. Others use an asterisk * to represent any number of letters, including zero. Thus, **edema* would retrieve *edema*, *oedema*, *lymphedema* and *lymphoedema*.

A trickier problem arises when completely different terms, rather than variants in spelling, are used to refer to the same concept. Consider another term from our question about employment among stroke survivors. *Stroke* can also be referred to as *cerebrovascular accident, cerebral vascular accident,* or *CVA*. One way to deal with this is to use the Boolean operator 'OR'. To search for articles that include the concept of *stroke* described using any of these terms, string them together like this:

stroke OR cerebrovascular accident OR cerebral vascular accident OR CVA

This search will return articles which include the concept of stroke if it is referred to by one or more of these terms.

An alternative to this approach is to use 'subject headings'. All the articles in CINAHL have been assigned subject headings – descriptors that describe the contents of the article. These make searching easier because once you identify a subject heading that describes the concept you are searching for, the specific terms used to describe it in the article do not matter. Once you find the most appropriate subject headings, you will be able to use them to find other relevant material.

It is not always easy to guess what term has been selected as the subject heading for your concept of interest. Most databases that use subject headings make them easier to find by offering the option to map your search terms to a subject heading. Mapping helps you to find the subject headings that are used in the database by automatically checking for the most appropriate one for your search term. For example, if you type 'stroke' as your search term and click the option to map your search term to a subject heading, CINAHL will return the page shown in Figure 4.5.

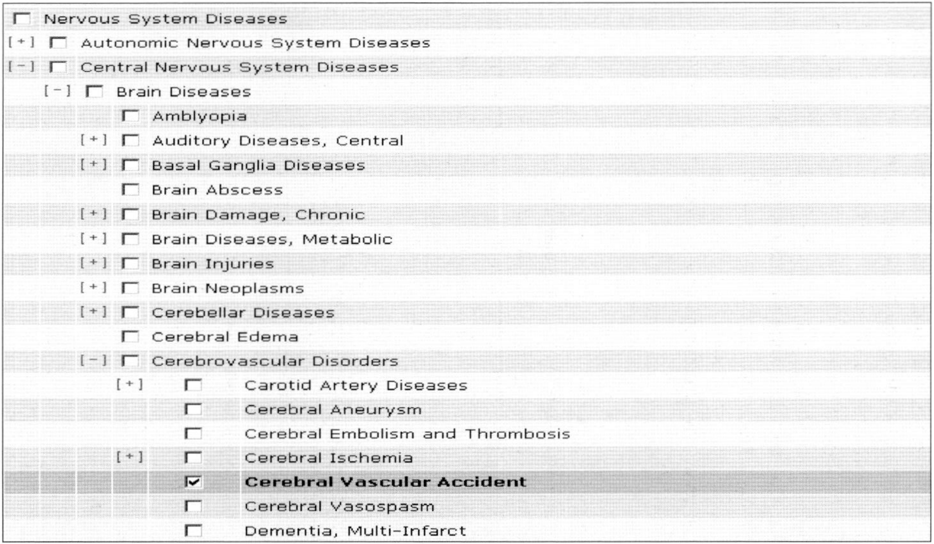

Fig. 4.5 Type 'stroke' as your search term and click the option to map your search term to a subject heading. CINAHL will return the page shown here.

This offers you the chance to see what CINAHL uses as the subject heading for the search term you entered. It also shows you where this subject heading fits in a hierarchy. Sometimes this alerts you to the fact that you are also interested in other, closely aligned concepts – perhaps *cerebral ischaemia* in this example – which you might also choose to search for. Or perhaps you would like a more- or less-encompassing subject heading, which can be found further up or down the hierarchy, respectively.

EFFICIENCY TIP NO. 3: READ A REVIEW ARTICLE If you are interested in a very popular research topic, you may find that even your most-focussed search strategy returns a large amount of relevant material. One way to cut down the amount of time you need to answer your question is to read one paper that reviews all the research that has been performed on the topic, instead of reading each individual piece of research. Whatever the question you might have in mind, a review can be designed to answer it. Unfortunately, not every question that may interest you will have had a review performed to answer it. Conversely, more than one review has been published for some questions.

You might reasonably expect that several reviews tackling the same question would reach the same conclusion. This is not always true because authors use a variety of methods to review the literature. Some methods create greater potential for bias to influence the results. To use your reading time efficiently and to avoid gaining a false impression of what the literature shows, you should read the review with the least potential for bias.

What types of bias can influence the results of a review? The first group of biases are not the fault of the reviewer. They all relate to whether and how the original studies are reported.

Some trials are performed but never get published – this is also called *file-drawer bias*. Unfortunately, it is not just a random set of trials that are not published; it is far more likely to be trials with negative or non-significant results. So this systematically skews the set of readily available trials, making your treatment look more favourable than it really is. *Time lag bias* is similar – the trials with statistically non-significant or negative results get published but it takes longer. Often reviewers only report those trials published in English, which again you might think is just eliminating a random couple of trials. Trials with significant outcomes are also, however, more likely to be published in English, creating a *language bias* for reviews that only consider English-language trials. The study authors might also choose to report only those outcomes that were significant, even though many others were measured. Thus, a *reporting bias* can be established.

Although reviewers do not cause these biases, there are steps that they can take in the conduct of the review to reduce them. The remaining sources of potential bias are directly related to the methods used by the reviewers.

Just as you might use electronic databases to search for trials, authors reviewing the literature do so as well. *Retrieval bias* relates to electronic searches. Trials can be coded differently in different databases and a search strategy that isn't tailored to each database may miss some trials. Also, if all the relevant databases are not searched, trials can be missed. If the reviewers include poor-quality trials with potentially biased results, the results of the review can be biased. This could be termed *quality bias.* Finally, there is the reviewer's *personal bias.* Whether conscious or subconscious, it is possible for reviewers to put their personal slant on the presentation of the results of a review. This could occur if, for example, some trials are given more prominence in the discussion or some relevant trials are not discussed at all.

A high-quality review is one which has eliminated as many of these sources of potential bias as possible. Table 4.1 shows the steps that can be taken to eliminate or minimise the potential for each bias to influence the results of the review.

The last strategy in Table 4.1 – pre-specifying a protocol and conducting the review according to that protocol – deserves further discussion. If the review is of high quality, the protocol will specify the other strategies listed in Table 4.1. Even if very few of the strategies are implemented, the very existence of a protocol is reassuring. Reviewers who are free to retrieve and include trials and to analyse the results in any way can choose a method that provides a result that satisfies their personal bias. Those who follow a protocol, however, have a means of circumventing such bias. Reviews that are conducted according to a protocol are termed 'systematic reviews'.

SEARCHING COCHRANE REVIEWS EFFICIENTLY

Of course, it is possible to design a protocol and then not follow it. Publishing the protocol for a review makes the reviewers accountable. This is standard practice for

TABLE 4.1   STRATEGIES FOR MINIMISING SOURCES OF BIAS IN A LITERATURE REVIEW

Sources of bias	Minimisation strategies
File-drawer bias and Time-lag bias	Ask researchers and expert clinicians in the field if they know of any relevant, unpublished trials. Check trial registers for unpublished trials. Check conference abstract books for otherwise unpublished trials. Contact researchers of any known unpublished trials to ask for unpublished data.
Language bias	Translate foreign-language trials.
Reporting bias	Request any unpublished data from authors.
Retrieval bias	Search all relevant databases. Use all relevant search terms.
Quality bias	Include only trials with minimal potential for bias.
Personal bias	Devise a protocol before commencing the review that defines how the review will be conducted, including: the search strategy the criteria for including studies, and the method of statistical analysis of the results. Conduct the review according to this protocol.

all systematic reviews done through the Cochrane Collaboration. Systematic reviews performed by members of the Cochrane Collaboration are published on an electronic database called the Cochrane Database of Systematic Reviews. This can be found at: www.mrw. interscience.wiley.com/cochrane/cochrane_clsysrev_ articles_fs.html.

All the systematic reviews on the Cochrane Database of Systematic Reviews have protocols that are published before the review is commenced. The protocols have expert editorial input and are carefully devised to eliminate as many sources of bias as possible. The pre-publication allows interested parties to suggest ways the protocol could be improved, as well as making the reviewers accountable to the final version. In addition, the Cochrane Collaboration provides their reviewers with the resources to hand search conference abstract books, have articles translated, and so on. All this makes the systematic reviews in the Cochrane Database of Systematic Reviews of high quality. Over 4000 systematic reviews have been published in the database and these are regularly updated. If you find one of these reviews that answers your question, you can expect a comprehensive and unbiased summary of the relevant, high-quality evidence.

Searching the Cochrane Database of Systematic Reviews is very simple. The titles of the reviews use a fairly standard format that mentions the intervention(s) being examined, the problem being treated, and the population in whom the intervention was trialled. For example, if you were interested in whether exercise was a useful strategy for combating osteoporosis in elderly women, you would expect it to be called something like

Exercise (INTERVENTION) for low bone density (PROBLEM) in elderly women (POPULATION). You could enter the intervention element, *exercise*, as a search term, as shown in Figure 4.6.

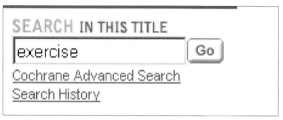

Fig. 4.6 Example search in the Cochrane Database of Systematic Reviews. (Reproduced with permission. Copyright John Wiley & Sons, Inc).

This retrieves a relevant review, entitled 'Exercise for preventing and treating osteoporosis in postmenopausal women' by Bonaiuti et al. (2002). It is difficult to find, however, among over 700 systematic reviews. A faster way than browsing the 700 is to try adding another search term to focus the search. If you add a term for the problem being treated, *bone density*, to your search terms, the retrieval narrows down to around 50 reviews. Even though we have not exactly matched the term from the title of the target review, the term *bone density* does appear in the abstract. Thus the target review still appears among the 50. This is a reasonable number of reviews to browse, so you browse the list and find the review you want.

Of course you may find excellent systematic reviews published outside the Cochrane Collaboration. You will have to examine carefully those reviews you retrieve with your searches, however, to determine whether they are systematic and whether the protocol has eliminated many sources of bias.

Reviews may not provide the whole answer

Reviews take time to perform, so they cannot include studies published between when the search was conducted and when the review was published. Thus, even the highest quality review is (at least theoretically) out-of-date by the time it is published. The greater the lag between a review's publication date and when you read it, the more important it is for you to check for subsequent studies. As mentioned above, some questions that arise in your clinical practice will not have been examined by a review. In this case, you will want to search for individual trials.

> **EFFICIENCY TIP NO. 4: STICK TO THE HIGHEST-QUALITY MATERIAL**   Just like the author of a high-quality systematic review, you do not want to pay attention to low-quality research because it is potentially biased. The general databases we have discussed so far do not discriminate between high- and low-quality research. It is very inefficient to have to trawl through the low-quality material to find what you want. If you are trying to answer a question about the efficacy of a therapy, you could instead search one of the discipline-specific databases that include only well-designed research. As an example, we will look at one of these databases, PED*ro*.

SEARCHING PED*ro* EFFICIENTLY

PED*ro* is the nickname for the Physiotherapy Evidence Database – a database of evidence about the effectiveness of physiotherapy interventions (Sherrington et al. 2000) PED*ro* is available at www.pedro.fhs.usyd. edu.au.

Two ways are available for searching PED*ro*: simple and advanced. A simple search checks all the fields for the search terms you have entered. An advanced search allows you to enter terms in specific fields, just like other databases. Thus, if you wished to find a trial by the author Parkinson, you could enter 'Parkinson' in the Author field. PED*ro* will then retrieve trials where one of the authors' names is Parkinson, but not all the trials about Parkinson's disease. An advanced search also allows you to select terms from pull-down menus for the following fields: Therapy, Problem, Body Part and Subdiscipline. As an example of how you might use these fields, suppose you were interested to know whether balance training helps prevent falls in the elderly. By selecting 'skill training' from the Therapy field, PED*ro* will retrieve trials which mention balance training, Cawthorne exercises, and so on. By selecting 'gerontology' from the Subdiscipline field, PED*ro* will retrieve trials where the average age of subjects is over 60 years. Thus entering terms as seen in Figure 4.7 would be a suitable advanced search.

Regardless of whether you perform a simple or an advanced search, there are several important features of the trials and reviews retrieved by PED*ro*. These features allow you to efficiently identify the highest quality source of evidence to answer your question, whether that be trials, a review, or a combination.

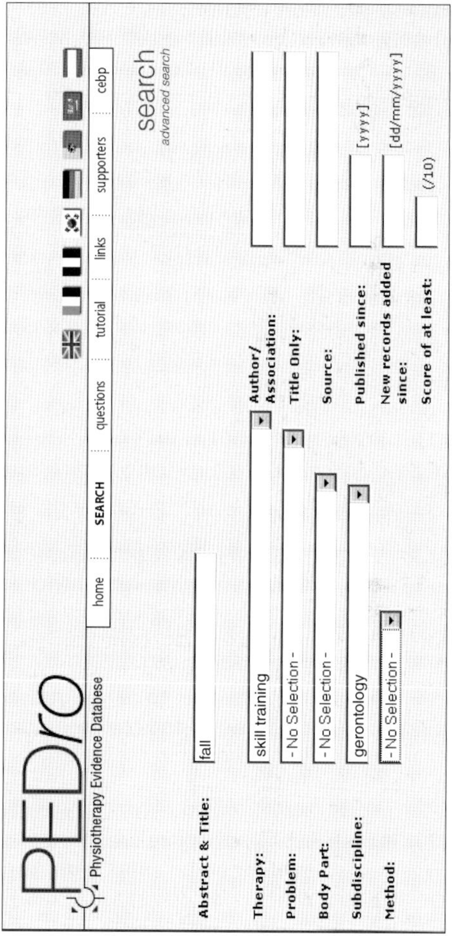

Fig. 4.7 Advanced search in PED*ro*.

Randomised trials on PEDro

First, all trials indexed on PEDro meet the criterion of having a randomised design. Randomised trials eliminate many sources of bias in their results. Searching with general databases, such as MEDLINE or CINAHL retrieves a mixture of randomised trials, unrandomised trials, epidemiological studies, case series and case reports, even if the 'clinical queries' filter is used. Because you want the highest-quality evidence about the effects of an intervention, you need to sift through and find the randomised trials. This is not always obvious from the titles or even from the abstracts. PEDro has already done this work for you, allowing you to hone in on the randomised trials.

Although all trials on PEDro meet a minimum criterion of quality by being randomised, other features of their design are considered to be quality criteria as well. As an example, imagine a trial where participants are randomised to either a treatment group or a control group that receives no treatment. The researcher who determines whether subjects are eligible for inclusion in this trial may be kept unaware of each upcoming group allocation on the random list. That is, the random allocation list is concealed. Why would a research team bother to keep this information from the researcher enrolling participants? If the researcher were aware, the decision about whether or not to include a person in a trial could be influenced by that awareness. This could produce systematic biases in otherwise random allocation. There is evidence that trials that keep the researchers unaware of the allocation list find more modest treatment effects (Schulz et al. 1995). This and other aspects of trial design are considered quality criteria because they can affect how biased the results could be. Once trials are indexed on PED*ro*, they are rated against a set of these quality criteria (Maher et al. 2003). When you search PED*ro*, the trials retrieved are listed with the trials meeting the highest number of these criteria first. This directs you to those trials with the highest likelihood of being valid and interpretable.

Another feature of the trials on PED*ro* is that all are to do with physiotherapy interventions. Thus, unlike the search results of a general database, you do not have to wade through articles related to medical, surgical or other interventions. Although you can specify the intervention somewhat with your search terms, this is not always effective. For example, suppose that you are interested in whether quadriceps exercises are beneficial after anterior cruciate ligament reconstruction. In this case, the patient population is defined by having had a surgical procedure. This makes it extremely difficult to enter a search term that does not also retrieve articles in which the surgical procedure itself is trialled or reviewed. The search term *ACL reconstruction* can be entered in PED*ro* without this headache, returning only articles examining physiotherapy interventions for this post-surgical population.

Systematic reviews on PED*ro*

The reviews indexed on PED*ro* all also meet certain criteria. Every review must contain a description of the methods used to perform the review. Also, the review must include at least one randomised clinical trial of a physiotherapy intervention.

When PED*ro* returns the results of your search, the systematic reviews are listed before the randomised trials. This directs you to the most efficient source of information first – summarised information. By examining the reviews, their thoroughness, and the year that their literature search was performed, you can make a decision about which other trials to read to supplement the information provided by the best review.

Depending on the search you perform, PED*ro* may also retrieve evidence-based clinical practice guidelines. Clinical practice guidelines are documents that:

- Systematically identify and examine the evidence related to a particular clinical condition
- Distil the evidence into key recommendations for patient management, and
- State how much evidence there is in support of each recommendation.

You can think of them as systematic reviews that answer more than a single question. They attempt to determine the evidence for how a disease or a major aspect of it should be managed. The guidelines indexed on PED*ro* also meet similar criteria to those that are applied to the systematic reviews. Answering your question with guidelines requires less time than reading each individual piece of research.

CONCLUSION

There are several reasons why you need to search efficiently for high-quality evidence about interventions. The health-related literature is too extensive to read everything. The high-quality evidence is arbitrarily located. Even simple searching of general databases retrieves a mixture of high- and low-quality material, making the best evidence time-consuming to find. The strategies and resources described in this chapter will provide you with the means to find, identify and read high-quality evidence efficiently. You should familiarise yourself with these databases and their features. Practise using them to develop your skills in searching efficiently.

LEARNING OUTCOMES

After reading this chapter you should have a basic understanding of . . .
- How to decide what to read
- How to search Journals
- How to search MEDLINE
- How to search CINAHL
- How to search Cochrane
- How to search PED*ro*.

REFERENCES

Bonaiuti D, Cranney A, Iovine R et al. 2002 Exercise for preventing and treating osteoporosis in postmenopausal women. Cochrane Database System Reviews 2.

Herbert R D, Maher C G, Moseley A M, Sherrington C 2001 Effective physiotherapy. British Medical Journal 323:788–790.

Maher C, Sherrington C, Herbert R, Moseley A, Elkins M 2003 Reliability of the PED*ro* scale for rating quality of randomized controlled trials. Physical Therapy 83:713–721.

Miser W F 1999 Critical appraisal of the literature. Journal of the American Board of Family Practice 12:315–333.

Moseley A M, Herbert R D, Sherrington C, Maher C G 2002 Evidence for physiotherapy practice: a survey of the physiotherapy evidence database (PED*ro*). Australian Journal of Physiotherapy 48:43–49.

Schulz K, Chalmers I, Hayes R, Altman D 1995 Empirical evidence of bias: dimensions of methodological quality associated with estimates of treatment effects in controlled trials. Journal of the American Medical Association 273:408–412.

Sherrington C, Herbert R D, Maher C G, Moseley A M 2000 PED*ro*. A database of randomized trials and systematic reviews in physiotherapy. Manual Therapy 5:223–226.

CHAPTER FIVE

Research ethics

Hugh Davies

THE VALUE OF RESEARCH AND MISDEMEANOURS IN THE CONDUCT OF RESEARCH

It is self-evident that medical treatments have improved in recent centuries and a cogent argument can be made that these developments are founded on the rise of empirical observation and experimentation from the

TABLE 5.1   ADVANCES AND MISDEMEANOURS IN MEDICAL RESEARCH

Examples of therapeutic advances over 300 years	Examples of misdemeanours in medical research
The introduction of Peruvian bark (quinine).	Human blood transfusions in the seventeenth century.
The introduction of smallpox inoculation.	Introduction of smallpox inoculation through experiments on prisoners.
The treatment of scurvy.	Development of an anti-syphilis serum.
The development of smallpox vaccination.	The Tuskegee experimental programme.
The establishment of anti septic techniques.	Experiments in Willowbrooke: From 1963 to 1966, children admitted to Willowbrooke, New York State School for the mentally defective were deliberately infected with the Hepatitis A virus to test the effect of a treatment; gamma globulin injections.
The discovery of penicillin.	Modern evidence of unethical research.
The identification of *H. pylori* as a cause of peptic ulcer disease.	

(Beecher 1966)

seventeenth century onwards. Consequently, our health and that of future generations depends on the health of medical research, which itself depends on our continuing trust and participation in medical trials.

While the ethical standing of most work remains unquestioned, there have been examples of unethical research in the past and there are good reasons to believe that the problem will continue. Research is, after all, no more than a human endeavour and susceptible to all the human failures. While it is therefore crucial that research continues, we, the subjects of research or members of the community, must be in a position to trust the researchers and their work.

The role of research ethics committees is: to contribute to the maintenance of public trust in research.

THE MODERN RESEARCHER'S ENVIRONMENT

The World Medical Association in its Declaration of Helsinki (a crucial reference for anyone reviewing or undertaking research) states in paragraph B13:

The design and performance of each experimental procedure involving human subjects should be clearly formulated in an experimental protocol. This protocol should be submitted for consideration, comment, guidance, and where appropriate, approval to a specially appointed ethical review committee, which must be independent of the investigator, the sponsor or any other kind of undue influence. This independent committee should be in conformity with the laws and regulations of the country in which the research experiment is performed. The committee has the right to monitor ongoing trials. The researcher has the obligation to provide monitoring information to the committee, especially any serious adverse events.

The researcher should also submit to the committee, for review, information regarding funding, sponsors, institutional affiliations, other potential conflicts of interest and incentives for subjects.

In the UK, this is reflected in the Royal College of Physicians report 'Guidelines on the practice of Ethics Committees in Medical Research involving Human Subjects':

It is now generally agreed that:

    (i)   *Research investigation on human subjects should conform with codes such as . . . Declaration of Helsinki . . .*

    (ii) *Investigators should not be the sole judges of whether their research does so conform.*

Both researchers and society now broadly accept this stipulation and in the UK, this is delegated to Research Ethics Committees (RECs); independent advisory committees of whom one-third of its membership must be people independent of the NHS and not conducting any research. Their role is to protect the dignity, rights, safety and well-being of participants but also to recognise the value of research.

ETHICS AND RESEARCH ETHICS

In a short text such as this, it is inappropriate to embark upon a lengthy discussion on the definition of 'research ethics', so for this chapter, I am going to define it as 'the analysis of research to determine what might be seen as fair and acceptable to the community in which the research is conducted'.

The study of research ethics therefore has purpose. It provides a framework that allows us to analyse our own beliefs in this field; explore how they fit into established models and make objective comparisons with those of others. It can help RECs reach a collective decision and promote fair, objective debate and decision-making.

For researchers, it can help them see their work from 'the patients' point of view'. It can help them assess the consequences for participants and determine whether the project would be fair and acceptable to those people.

ETHICAL FRAMEWORKS

Research ethics can be seen to be based upon 'ethical frameworks' that lay a foundation for the ethical analysis of research. It is important however to understand these are no more than a means of analysing a research proposal. They are not mutually exclusive and one does not have moral superiority. When they lead to different conclusions, it is often a matter of fine judgement, which should predominate. Many such frameworks exist and this plethora can confuse the student. The two commonest approaches are:

1. The consequentialist approach.

2. The rule or principle-based approach.

1. The consequentialist approach

This assesses the ethical value of research by its *outcome* rather than its *content* or *procedure*. An acceptable (ethical) project would be one that produces net benefit over cost and it therefore allows for a cost or ethical infringements but expects these to be minimised to ensure the outcome is beneficial.

2. *The rule or principle-based approach*

In contrast to the consequentialist approach, this assesses the ethical worth of research by the processes involved. It is about doing what is right and by extension, not doing what is wrong.

In biomedical ethics, the most widely known set of ethical principles are those described by Beauchamp and Childress (2001).

- The Principle of Beneficence: we have a duty to do good, to benefit others
- The Principle of Non-Maleficence: we have a duty to avoid harming others
- The Principle of Respect for Autonomy: we have a duty to allow others to make decisions for themselves
- The Principle of Justice: we must treat others equally.

An idea for research

As part of a PhD in physiotherapy, Eddie Kingsley plans to complete a research project.

On one of her attachments to a children's chest unit in the USA, she was interested to hear about a new chest physiotherapy technique called 'chuffing' to clear lung secretions.

When she undertook her clinical attachment at a similar unit in the UK, the children often told her that standard therapy took too much time and they didn't do it!

She had the idea that chuffing might help.

Moral or ethical consideration is not a 'bolt on' or 'optional extra'; it is central to the development of a research proposal

Moral deliberation can rarely, if ever, be absolute and you may need to reason to reach a judgement. These reasons are as important as your conclusions. If you have reasoned you will be able to reach a conclusion and it is more than likely that you will have reached a fair decision. Be prepared to explain your reasons as justification.

Present your views with honesty, but with the possibility there may be other ways to see the problem. Moral vacillation may only suggest to a reviewer that you have no perception of how your subjects will feel.

Anticipate and discuss ethical issues. Engage in the debate, if you propose to conduct a piece of research, you cannot sit on the fence! This goes back to the idea that you need to look at the project through your subject's eyes.

Practically, meet deadlines; this will ease the passage of your proposal, and indicate that you have a responsible and 'professional' attitude and even when you disagree with the reviewer, exercise restraint. Reviewers *may* have a point, and you lose much if the debate becomes hostile, even if you are right. The value of research ethics is that it can provide an objective analysis of a project and allow easier dialogue and the marginalisation of prejudice. Pragmatically, there are avenues for complaint through the National Research Ethics Service.

From the very beginning, the researcher should look at their ideas from the point of view of potential subjects and ask (and answer) the questions. Patients or patient groups could be asked for their opinion and ideas:

- Is it fair to ask them to participate?
- What extra demands will be imposed upon them?
- To what risks (if any) will they be exposed?
- How will they see and experience this project and what will it mean for them?
- Are they given a fair chance to decide whether they wish to participate and is the choice offered a true choice?
- Will it benefit my patients?

A researcher also needs to explore the value of the project.

Why am I asking this (research) question?

Does it require an answer, will it improve practice, add to our knowledge of the condition or develop my clinical and research skills. All are worthy objectives, but it is important to recognise that much research will not have such immediate purpose. It will, however, help persuade reviewers of its ethical value.

Has it been answered before?

All research should be founded on what is currently known, and a 'review of the literature' is a crucial preparatory step. The question may have been addressed already, and such reading might give guidance on the best method of research. It is not necessarily unethical to ask the same question, but review of the literature may suggest the best way to frame it.

Is it worth answering?

This will emerge from the review of the literature but may also require discussion with current practitioners and patient groups.

Will the project answer the question?

Once the purpose of the research is defined and a clear question is posed, it is vital to ask whether your proposal will be able to answer it. This will require a critical appraisal of all aspects of methodology and (in the case of quantitative work) statistical advice.

PRACTICAL ASPECTS
A review of a research project in the UK

HOW MIGHT SUCH APPROACHES BE APPLIED TO EDDIE'S PROJECT?

As part of a PhD in physiotherapy, Eddie Kingsley plans to complete a research project.

She had the idea that the physiotherapy technique of 'chuffing' might help children with cystic fibrosis.

THE CONSEQUENTIALIST APPROACH

Eddie would argue that determining the better treatment will benefit children with cystic fibrosis. There may be theoretical reasons for this. Chuffing is quicker and therefore more easily fitted into a child's day.

But if standard physiotherapy has been found to be effective, some children may be given inferior treatment (chuffing) in a comparative study. However, once the better treatment is determined and results

Continued

published, all children with cystic fibrosis can receive the more effective treatment. For this argument it does not matter which treatment is better.

Such issues as the need for consent would be judged on its effect on the trial. If, for example, certain groups might not consent and consequently jeopardise the results of the trial it would be deemed unethical to ask for consent.

THE RULE OR PRINCIPLE-BASED APPROACH

The first two principles would demand that Eddie and the medical community felt the two treatments were equally effective. If not, she would be harming those allocated to the inferior treatment and infringing her duty to do what is best for our patients (beneficence) and avoid harming them (non-maleficence). These objections might be met if the inferiority were explained and the families and children, for altruistic reasons, took on the study, although this places respect for autonomy above the duties of beneficence and non-maleficence. It would at least demand that Eddie was certain the families and children fully understood the decision they were making.

Consent would be central to the respect for a patient's autonomy. Parents are expected to make decisions for their children until they themselves are competent to do so.

THE REMIT OF RESEARCH ETHICS COMMITTEES

The Governance Arrangements for RECs (GAfREC) stipulates that:

3.1.   . . . any research proposal involving:

a. *patients and users of the NHS. This includes all potential research participants recruited by virtue of the patient or user's past or present treatment by, or use of, the NHS. It includes NHS patients treated under contracts with private sector institutions*

b. *individuals identified as potential research participants because of their status as relatives or carers of patients and users of the NHS, as defined above*

c. *access to data, organs or other bodily material of past and present NHS patients*

d. *foetal material and IVF involving NHS patients*

e. *the recently dead in NHS premises*

f. *the use of, or potential access to, NHS premises or facilities*

g. *NHS staff – recruited as research participants by virtue of their professional role must be reviewed by an REC. Audit and service evaluation are excluded.*

Nevertheless, all healthcare activity will raise ethical issues. This policy is not in itself founded on ethical deliberations, rather on a decision on where the responsibility for ethical review should be placed.

If we were to consider Eddie's research project, where should the responsibility lie – with Eddie, her supervisor, the academic institution, the hospital or an independent REC?

What does this mean practically for Eddie?

Clearly it will involve NHS patients (*3.1.a* above) but *is it research?* Use Table 5.2 to draw you own conclusions.

TABLE 5.2　SUMMARIES OF RESEARCH, AUDIT AND SERVICE/THERAPY EVALUATION

Research	Audit	Service/therapy evaluation
Motivated to generate new knowledge.	Motivated to provide best care.	Motivated to define current care.
Quantitative research: is hypothesis based. Qualitative research: explores themes following established methodology.	Designed to answer the question: 'Does this service reach a predetermined standard?' Measures against a standard.	Designed to answer the question: 'What standard does this service achieve?' Measures current service without reference to a standard.
May involve a new treatment.	Does not involve a new treatment.	Does not involve a new treatment.
May involve additional therapies or investigations.	Involves no more than administration of questionnaire or record analysis.	Involves no more than administration of questionnaire or record analysis.
May involve allocation to treatment groups *not* chosen by HCP or patient.	Does not involve allocation to treatment groups: the HCP and patients choose.	Does not involve allocation to treatment groups: the HCP and patients choose.
May involve randomisation.	Does *not* involve randomisation.	Does *not* involve randomisation.

TABLE 5.2 SUMMARIES OF RESEARCH, AUDIT AND SERVICE/THERAPY EVALUATION *cont.*		
Research	**Audit**	**Service/therapy evaluation**
Although any of these three may raise ethical problems, under current guidance:		
Requires REC review	Does not require REC review	Does not require REC review
HCP, healthcare professional.		

The Research Ethics Committee application form

Applicants to the National Research Ethics Committee must complete and submit the REC application form. It is this and the patient information sheets that inform the committee, as not all receive a copy of the research protocol. If you have written a research protocol, this should present few problems. It might be suggested that this could be the structure for your research protocol. See:

http://www.corec.org.uk/applicants/apply/docs/Blank_Form_ (reference_only).pdf

Many questions request straightforward information such as the title of the project (QA1), the researcher (QA2) and how long the study will last (QA3). Listed below with exploratory text, are questions that look at the ethics of the application.

As part of a PhD in physiotherapy, Eddie Kingsley wishes to complete a research project.

Eddie proposes that chuffing will slow the usual decline of lung function that is seen in children with cystic fibrosis. Having taken statistical advice and knowing the standard deviation of lung function measurements and their normal rate of decline in this group, it is recognised that she requires a study of 80 children randomised 1:1 to either chuffing or standard physiotherapy. The children need to be followed for 2 years.

The project has been reviewed by the National Children's Cystic Fibrosis Interest Group, who have provided favourable scientific critique and are in full support. They conclude with:

The problems of compliance with physiotherapy and its efficacy are unanswered and this study will make a contribution to the scientific basis of physiotherapy in children with cystic fibrosis. It is felt the design is practical and will answer the question posed. Support and facilities are adequate for the project.

MEASUREMENTS
Standard lung function tests will be undertaken at 3-monthly intervals, as is routine clinical practice. The study will *not* impose any extra burden on parents or children.

SUBJECTS
A total of 240 children with cystic fibrosis attend the clinic and discussion with the clinicians indicates it would be feasible to recruit the requisite number within 3 months.

RECRUITMENT
Physicians will explain the study and give out an information sheet. If the families wish to enrol, they will be asked to ring the researcher and an appointment will be made to provide a full explanation and go through the recruitment process.

CONSENT
This will be sought by one physiotherapist (EK). The study will be explained to both parents and children. Appropriate information sheets have been designed for children aged 5–10 and 11–16 and their parents.

INCLUSION CRITERIA
Children between the ages of 8 and 12 for whom physiotherapy is a standard part of treatment.

EXCLUSION CRITERIA
CONFIDENTIALITY
All data will be anonymised by allocation of a study number. Only EK will hold the key, to be stored in a locked filing cabinet in the department.

REVIEW OF POTENTIAL HAZARDS AND RESEARCH COMMITMENT
Harm
The children will receive nothing above standard treatment and no harm is anticipated. Records will be held confidentially as above.

SAMPLES
None will be collected.

Questions A7–10, A18, A46, A47: the purpose of the study, the question being posed, the study methodology and the ability of the study to answer it

Many, if not most, committees take a consequentialist view of a proposal, asking themselves 'What is the worth of this research, what is its purpose, what 'gap' in knowledge will it fill or how will it contribute to healthcare?' This includes the development of research expertise. While a project with no immediate purpose is not in itself unethical, a committee persuaded of purpose is likely to take a more favourable view.

For an applicant, it is therefore important to provide a clear, realistic assessment of the purpose of the study. The ends, however, cannot justify all the means. This consequentialist approach needs to be balanced with the recognition that researching healthcare professionals have duties to their patients/participants. The REC represents the patients and seeks to see a project from their point of view.

Questions A11–17: research procedures

When assessing the balance of risk and benefit of a study as well as what might be termed the 'burden of the project (what it involves for the subject)', the committee needs to know the routine procedures the subjects will undergo; those that are in addition to such routine clinical practice and are part of the study protocol and procedures that will be withheld. Simple explanation is essential and a picture or diagram may be worth a thousand words.

Consider the 'Stick it on the fridge test': Could participants put a flow chart or diagram on their fridge door to remind them what they need to do and where they need to be?

Risk needs to be carefully considered and if there is concern, consult your patient groups. If there *is* benefit, it should be outlined but not used as false inducement.

Questions A20–21: recruitment of subjects

Many different methods may be used: internet, television, radio, advertisement or information through a clinical encounter. At this stage, there should be few, if any, therapeutic promises. There should also be no coercion or unacceptable inducement and information collected should be the minimum required to explain the study. RECs will look carefully at the relationship between the potential subject and the 'recruiter', to ensure the subject is not beholden in any way that might influence their decision. Identification of potential subjects by exploration of medical records should only be conducted by a member of the clinical team.

Questions A22–23: inclusion and exclusion criteria

No one should be unfairly excluded from or included in research. Such actions (both inclusion and exclusion) therefore need justification. This could be depicted as in Table 5.3.

Mirkin (1975) has deliberated on the consequences of therapy with and without prior trials. He concludes:

This policy reflects a choice made between two undesirable outcomes: Society may choose to forbid a drug evaluation . . . This choice would certainly reduce the risk of

TABLE 5.3   THE RISKS AND BENEFITS OF INCLUSION AND EXCLUSION IN TRIALS

	Risk	Benefit
Inclusion	Risk: Of research procedures or withholding standard procedure Of new therapy Of intrusion To confidentiality Of a change of relationship with the HCP: the researcher's and clinician's goals may not overlap completely.	Researchers usually believe that a new treatment they are testing will be better than an existing or lack of treatment. The biggest benefit of medical research is often not directly to the person involved, but is the increase in medical knowledge that benefits future patients. While taking part in a study, your general health may be monitored closely by the researchers.
Exclusion	Belonging to an under-researched group (e.g. children or women) Continuing use of dangerous therapy Continuing use of ineffective therapy Continuing use of incorrect dosages Stagnant or inappropriate healthcare	No research procedures No potentially inferior new therapy No intrusion No risk to confidentiality No change of relationship with HCP

HCP, healthcare professional.

damaging individuals through research. However, this would maximise the possibility of random disaster resulting from the use of inadequately investigated drugs. In the final analysis it seems safe to predict that more individuals would be damaged; however the damage would be distributed randomly rather than imposed upon preselected individuals.

Question A24: will the participants be from any of the following groups? (there follows a list of 'vulnerable groups')

- Children under 16
- Adults with learning disabilities
- Adults who are unconscious or very severely ill
- Adults who have a terminal illness
- Adults in emergency situations
- Adults with mental illness (particularly if detained under Mental Health Legislation); adults suffering from dementia
- Prisoners; young offenders
- Adults in Scotland who are unable to consent for themselves
- Healthy volunteers
- Those who could be considered to have a particularly dependent relationship with the investigator, e.g. those in care homes, medical students
- Other vulnerable groups.

This list is so large, it may be thought that everybody is 'vulnerable'! It is perhaps better to ask: 'Could any potential subject be unable to represent their interests or be susceptible to coercion?'

If so, you must pay greater attention to the question: 'How do you propose to ensure consent is valid?'

- The subject or his representative should understand the information presented
- The choice must be realistic
- Participation should be voluntary and free of undue influence.

Question A25: multiple studies

Concern is often expressed about subjects participating in more than one research project and committees sometimes consider the burden of participation in more than one trial, but limited published evidence suggests this is not a concern to patients. Certainly, subjects should not be recruited to a study if they are already in one and:

1. Recruitment would compromise patient safety.

2. Such inclusion would undermine the scientific basis of either study.

Questions A26–28: consent

Obtaining the subject's permission to undertake a research project is seen to recognise the autonomy of the individual – to decide for himself what they will do. Such respect for autonomy is central to much current ethical opinion and if research is to be undertaken without consent, a clear justification will be required.

For consent to be valid, the potential participant must be 'competent' and provided with adequate information (what a reasonable person in such a situation would expect).

A competent person will:

- Understand in simple language what the medical treatment is, its purpose and nature and why it is being proposed
- Understand its principal benefits, risks and alternatives (in research it is also important for the subject to understand possible *lack* of benefits)
- Understand in broad terms what will be the consequences of not receiving the proposed treatment
- Retain the information long enough to make an effective decision
- Make a free choice.

The decision must be voluntary and the potential participant must be free of duress.

It is expected the potential participant will be given information both verbally and in the form of a patient information sheet. Information about writing a patient information sheet can be found on the NRES website.

When the subjects may not be competent to provide valid consent, the committee may wish to know who will have the task of assessing competence and what training they have had.

Supporting views – World Medical Association Declaration of Helsinki:

22.

In any research on human beings, each potential subject must be adequately informed of the aims, methods, sources of funding, any possible conflicts of interest, institutional affiliations of the researcher, the anticipated benefits and potential risks of the study and the discomfort it may entail. The subject should be informed of the right to abstain from participation in the study or to withdraw consent to participate at any time without reprisal. After ensuring that the subject has understood the information, the physician should then obtain the subject's freely given informed consent, preferably in writing. If the consent cannot be obtained in writing, the non-written consent must be formally documented and witnessed.

Obtaining consent is central to the Department of Health (UK) policy on treatment and research. The Medical Research Council (2001) have stated:

Researchers can only proceed if they have obtained voluntary informed consent from the participant to participate in research. Special safeguards apply when this is not possible.

Question A29: participants who may have difficulties in adequate understanding of English

This question is asked to consider how such subjects would be recruited and managed. Disease patterns and health needs in the ethnic minorities are under-researched and consequently, such groups may be excluded from the benefits of research.

If trials closely follow clinical care, there is little reason to argue against recruitment. Any clinical care in such patients will require an interpreter who can be used to help treatment and research. If this is not undertaken, the researcher must explain why translations will not be available.

In studies of access to services, researchers must justify exclusion of those with limited English, as these are the very subjects likely to have difficulties using healthcare resources. This group has a special need to be included in research into health services and their exclusion in such studies must be seriously questioned.

Research involving such groups needs methodological consideration as well. Frequently used and well established questionnaires are likely to have been validated in languages other than English, but lesser known ones may not. This might question their validity. Quantitative tests may have different normal ranges.

Questions A33–34: payments to subjects
Payments are permitted. Subjects should not be out of pocket if they participate in research, but they should not be coercive, nor should subjects be paid on the basis of risk.

Questions A35–36: compensation
It would seem only fair that participants who suffer as a consequence of taking part in research should be recompensed. The explanation of such arrangements should be part of the process of obtaining consent and this information must be included in the Information Sheet.

Compensation for harm arising from negligence is normally the responsibility of the employer of the local researcher. When the NHS sponsors research, there is no provision to offer advance compensation for non-negligent harm to participants. A person suffering injury as a result of having taken part in research will need to pursue a claim for negligence through litigation, or may be offered an *ex gratia* payment by the Trust or Medical School. Each case will be considered on its merits.

It is essential that the researcher obtains management approval before starting a project, so as to ensure that the care organisation is aware of the possibility of a compensation claim should a problem occur. Separate cover for non-negligent harm for participants may be required in some circumstances. This will usually be covered by the ABPI guidelines for a drug trial, and by Health Service Guidelines for NHS sponsored research.

Questions A37–38: dissemination of results

If there is to be broader benefit from the research, positive and negative results need to be published. This recognises the subjects' contribution to a process that may offer no personal benefit.

Reviewers may therefore expect to see ways in which the project (not simply the results) will be placed in the public domain.

Questions A39–44: data handling and confidentiality

As with all healthcare activity, the researcher has a duty to handle participant information appropriately (in an ethical manner). It is important to recognise this does not imply absolute secrecy; rather confidentiality (there *may* be times when information needs to be disclosed without consent).

This is best covered by the 'Caldicott Principles', derived from the Caldicott report:

Principle 1: Justify the purpose(s) for obtaining the information.

Principle 2: Don't use person-identifiable information unless it is absolutely necessary.

Principle 3: Use the minimum necessary person-identifiable information.

Principle 4: Access to person-identifiable information should be on a strict need-to-know basis.

Principle 5: Everyone with access to person-identifiable information should be aware of their responsibilities.

Principle 6: Understand and comply with the law.

Questions A 48–53: statistical aspects of the research

An important question within consequentialist analysis is, 'Can the study answer the question?' Statistics are the numerical means by which this is done in quantitative studies. Qualitative studies can provide equally important conclusions but analysis will be methodologically different.

Questions A61–63: payment to researchers

The relationship between HCP and patient may change if the HCP participates in research. Any payment to a researcher should not be such that he or she might be tempted to fail to meet his or her duty of care.

Question A64: conflicts of interest

Most, if not all, ethics guidance stipulates that the well-being of the patient must be the primary concern of the healthcare professional (HCP), and payment or inducement that might undermine this must be declared and explored. The committee will need to be satisfied that such reward will not influence the researcher's behaviour or detract from his duty of care.

Question A67: end of trial arrangements

Some argue that participants should receive effective treatment determined by the study and that an experiment in which there was no commitment to provide effective therapy for all in the study would be using people as a means to the researcher's own end rather than an end in itself.

Guidance on this is unclear and in the end, it seems to be left to RECs to conclude case by case.

Therapeutic benefits of current trials may be marginal and it seems unlikely any trial will find a radical cure nowadays. Consequently, appropriate therapy emerges from consideration of many trials. The smaller therapeutic effect has other consequences: trials need to be larger and the statistical analysis more sophisticated. Both factors mean that many subjects finish a trial long before results are known.

Many therapies look at health maintenance (antihypertensives and blood sugar control are such examples) and therefore need to be conducted over a lengthy time period. Results are only available again after some time and any commitment to therapy would be for a prolonged period or even the life span.

In most countries, there is now a strict process of licensing that would make medical practitioners liable for adverse events if they prescribed unlicensed medications. Companies are prohibited from promoting medications for unlicensed use.

DECISIONS AVAILABLE TO A RESEARCH ETHICS COMMITTEE

Favourable
Provisional favourable opinion subject to Site Specific Assessment
Provisional opinion with request for further information

The assessment of such further information will be delegated to the chairman alone, chairman and one or more named members, a sub-committee meeting or, exceptionally, a full meeting.

No opinion

The committee was unable to reach a decision without consulting a specialist referee.

Unfavourable opinion

Where a REC has given an unfavourable opinion, the applicant may seek further review as follows:

- A new application may be submitted to the same REC, accommodating the REC's concerns. This is processed as a new application
- A second review of the same application may be obtained from another REC by giving notice of appeal to the National Research Ethics Service.

Notification of the decision is to be sent in writing within 10 working days of the meeting.

More details can be found on the National Research Ethics Service website.

INFORMATION SHEETS

It is now expected that researchers provide written information when obtaining consent to help the potential participant decide whether they want to take part. The level of detail should be appropriate to the nature of the study and the population to be studied. (Detailed guidance can be found on the NRES website.)

Such material should incorporate:

- Brief and clear information on the essential elements of the specific study
- What the research is about
- The condition or treatment under study
- The voluntary nature of involvement
- What will happen to the participant during and after the trial
- What usual treatment may be withheld
- The participant's responsibilities
- The potential risks
- Any inconvenience or restrictions balanced against the potential benefits (if any)
- Alternative management (in therapeutic trials).

This should allow the participant to make an initial choice of whether the study is of interest to them and they wish to read and discuss further.

Further details which should also be provided:

- Arrangements for confidentiality and data protection
- Communication with the GP
- Indemnity and compensation
- How the study will be placed in the public domain.

Information sheets should be written in simple, non-technical terms and be easily understood by a lay person. As a guide, the language level used should be no more difficult than that used in the information leaflets of medicines for the general public or in tabloid newspapers. The tone should be invitational and not coercive or overly persuasive. It is good practice to try out the information sheet on representatives of the group likely to be recruited and where possible, to involve representatives in the writing of the information sheet.

Information sheets for children (minors) and young people

It is recommended that information sheets are produced for the following age ranges, which broadly reflect cognitive stages of development.

- Children 5 years and under
- Children 6–12 years
- Children 13–15 years

and parents/guardians.

When designing information sheets for children, researchers need to consider:

- Their likely attention span
- Their potential fear of hospitals/procedures
- Their mental capacity if affected by disease
- Their disease severity
- Their previous experience of illness (some children have greater knowledge as the result of long-term illness, e.g. cystic fibrosis).

Ideally, such material should be shorter than that designed for adults.

It is good practice and will help to show your information sheets to a group of similar aged children to the study for comment, before you submit the formal version to the REC.

As with adults, child information sheets should accompany verbal explanations.

It is important to give guidelines in your information about how the study will affect the child at home, school and their social activities.

THE COLLECTION OF SAMPLES

The important role of obtaining and studying tissue samples in medical research is virtually universally accepted, and it is seen that such work must continue. The physical risks involved in donating most common samples (urine, saliva, blood) will usually be minimal. More invasive procedures (liver marrow or lung biopsy) require clearer justification. The consequences of analysis of the specimen must be considered, along with any consequences for the family.

General questions to consider:

- Do the benefits outweigh the risks?
- Are the risks less than minimal?
- Are the risks of taking the sample and its analysis clearly explained?

Under UK law, it is not legally possible to own human tissue. The MRC working party felt it was therefore more important to recognise 'Custodianship', the individual who has responsibility for safe storage, safeguarding the donor's interests and for the control of, use of, or disposal of the material. Samples should be regarded as a gift. It is deemed unethical for either party to derive profit from tissue itself, but it is accepted that profit can be made from developments made from the study of such samples. By *giving* tissue, the MRC working party felt that subjects could not expect to profit from donation.

Beyond the usual considerations around consent for research projects, potential subjects need to understand how the sample will be obtained; any risk; what the sample is to be used for; who will have access; how long it will be stored and whether future research projects may use the sample and how such projects will be reviewed.

Although 'blanket consent', i.e. 'samples could be used for any medical experiment' is not acceptable, it is accepted that subjects can be asked to consent to broadly defined research.

In *some* cases, consent may be unnecessary (quality assurance and some teaching), but this will require REC consideration. From an ethical stance, it would seem that consent might not be needed for:

- Health-related research on material from living people where the material is not linked to an identifiable individual and the research has been ethically approved (probably an REC)
- Proper conduct of treatment (audit, quality assurance, performance assessment)
- Necessary public health of the nation (public health monitoring, health-related education and training).

If consent is not sought, it is good practice to ensure that patients are informed that their samples may be used for research once all clinical requirements have been fulfilled.

Linkage of samples

Samples that are linked to demographic data provide a richer, more valuable resource. There is thus tension between scientific interests and the risk of breaching confidentiality.

Key principles are therefore suggested:

- It must be understood that personal information is confidential
- Research using identifiable patient data must be approved by an REC
- The minimal necessary amount of personal data should be used
- All personal information must be coded *as far and as early as possible*
- Subjects should be told what personal information will be stored and who might have access
- Personal data should only be divulged to people with an equal duty of confidentiality
- Principal investigators have a duty to ensure security is in place.

There are many classifications for samples; the MRC classification has received broad acceptance:

Anonymised samples or data have had any identifying information removed, such that it is not possible for the researcher using them to identify the individual to whom they relate.

Linked anonymised samples or data are fully anonymous to the people who receive or use them (e.g. the research team) but contain information or codes that would allow others (e.g. the clinical team who collected them or an independent body entrusted with safe-keeping of the code), to link them back to identifiable individuals.

Unlinked anonymised samples or data contain no information that could reasonably be used by anyone to identify the individuals who donated them or to whom they relate.

Coded samples or data have a coded identification to protect the confidentiality of the individual during routine use, but it is possible for the user to break the code and thus identify the individual from whom they were obtained.

DISCLOSURE OF RESULTS

Researchers must give consideration to disclosure of results before starting the study, and proposals should be put before the REC. Any decision will be influenced by:

- The possibility of benefit
- The possibility of harm
- Right to know balanced against the right *not* to know
- Consequences for family.

If practical, a clear distinction should be made between diagnostic testing and testing in medical research. If a research subject or their clinician later requests diagnostic services, a new specimen should be obtained. This should be explained to the research subject.

If the result of a test undertaken as part of a research protocol may be passed on to the participant or added to the medical record, then that patient must have been fully informed about the test(s) and prior specific consent sought.

Researchers need to be particularly aware of the public's sensitivity about genetic information. *All* consequences must be considered before the project is presented to an REC:

- Consequences for family members
- Employment issues
- Insurance issues
- 'Paternity' issues.

SURPLUS TISSUE

Such material might be considered to be 'abandoned'. It is recommended however, that individual consent should be obtained for the use for research of human material surplus to clinical requirements and that an ethics committee must approve all research using such human material. There must, however, be explicit separation of the consent to the treatment or diagnostic test from the consent to the use of surplus tissue for research.

At the very least, for example, patients should be made aware in any surgical consent form that they sign that surplus material may be used for research.

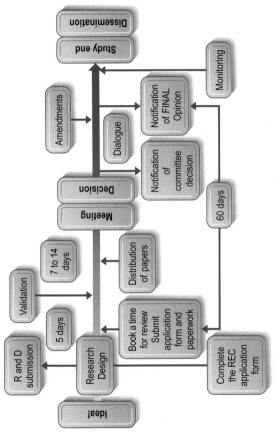

Figure 5.1 Timelines for ethical review of research.

LEARNING OUTCOMES

After reading this chapter you should have a basic
understanding of . . .

- Research & misdemeanours in the conduct of
  research
- Ethical frameworks
- The remit of Research Ethics Committees and the
  decisions available to them
- Information sheets, the collection of samples and
  disclosing results

REFERENCES

Beauchamp T L, Childress J F 2001 Principles of biomedical
ethics, 5th revised edn. Oxford University Press, USA.

Beecher H K 1966 Ethics and clinical research. New England
Journal of Medicine 274:1354–60.

Medical Research Council UK 2001 Human tissue and
biological samples for use in research. Online. Available:
http://www.mrc.ac.uk.

NRES (National Research Ethics Service) Online. Available:
www.nres.npsa.nhs.uk/.

CHAPTER SIX

Sampling, validity and reliability

Stuart Porter

Obviously, you cannot do your research project on everyone, so one thing you will need to think about is: who are you going to choose (your sample) and how are you going to choose them.

WHAT IS A SAMPLE?

A sample is a part of a statistical population whose properties we can investigate as a means of obtaining information about the properties of the whole.

Who makes up the sample?

A sample can be a group of people, patients' arms, legs, X-rays, drugs, diseases, etc.

WHY SAMPLE?

If we looked at the entire population, this would be a census. This sometimes has to be done but it is often

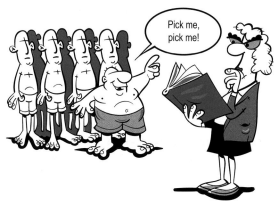

Fig. 6.1 A non-representative sample.

not practical in a research setting. Obviously, it is cheaper and quicker to observe a part of the population. But . . . there are risks with choosing a sample (see Fig. 6.1).

A sample is expected to mirror the population from which it comes; however, there is no guarantee that any sample will be precisely representative of the population from which it has been taken. For example, let us assume that you are curious about what it is like to undergo a hip replacement.

You know that all patients are different so they are likely to have different perceptions. You believe you must get access to these perceptions. You decide that you will conduct one-to-one interviews. The total number of people in the UK who have had hip replacements will be very large; so you know you cannot speak to all of them. For the type of information desired, a small wisely selected sample of patients can serve the purpose.

However, you need to ensure that the sample you choose is typical of the wider population. So you go through the files of all patients and select every 10th case to request for interview. A sample like the one above may provide you with needed information quickly.

Sampling: partly accessible populations

Some populations are so difficult to access or so small in number that only a small sample can ever be used, e.g. Siamese twins or those who have very rare genetic conditions.

Sampling: practical implications in industry and other testing procedures

Sampling may be useful when the nature of the observation is in itself destructive. Good examples of this occur in quality control. For example, to test the quality of medicines or food, to determine whether it is acceptable, some of it must be destroyed. It is of course not possible to destroy all of the food or medicine produced so, in this case, only a sample is used to assess the quality.

SELECTING A SAMPLE

Your choice of sampling procedure depends on its susceptibility to error; how practical it is and its cost. A chance component (sometimes called random error) will always be present no matter how carefully your sampling procedures have been implemented (i.e. your chances of picking the alien in Fig. 6.1). The only way to minimise chance sampling errors is to select a sufficiently large sample (sample 1000 humans and the odd alien does not matter as much – only 1/1000 of your sample is alien! But it you only choose three people and one of them is alien, then 33.3% of your sample is not typical).

TYPES OF SAMPLES
Convenience samples

A convenience sample results when the most convenient units are chosen from a population for observation. However, care should be taken, as the things or people who are most convenient to access may not be the best ones for your project. For example, it may be most convenient to stop students in the university corridor on a Friday afternoon to ask them about their study habits, but there may be a risk that only the most dedicated students are in the building on a Friday afternoon. Hence, any results that you obtained may be biased.

Random samples

A random sample allows a known probability that each unit will be chosen. It is sometimes referred to as a probability sample. Random numbers can be used and every member of the population has an equal chance of being selected; rather like rolling dice when there is an equal chance of scoring a 1, 2, 3, 4, 5 or 6.

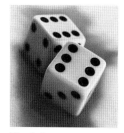

Fig. 6.2

Types of random samples
Simple random sampling

A simple random sample is obtained by choosing units in such a way that each unit in the population has an equal chance of being selected. Data collection can be made simpler by selecting every 10th or 100th uniform example after the first unit has been chosen randomly. This procedure is called systematic random sampling.

Systematic random sampling

A systematic random sample is obtained by selecting one unit on a random basis and choosing additional elementary units at evenly spaced intervals until the desired number of units is obtained. For example, there are 100 students in your physiotherapy class. You want a sample of 20 from these 100. If you are making use of systematic random sampling, divide 100 by 20. Randomly select any number between one and five. Suppose the number you have picked is three, that will be your starting number. So student No. 3 has been selected. From there you will select every fifth name until you reach the last one.

1, 2, **3,** 4, 5, 6, 7, **8,** 9, 10, 11, 12, **13,** 14, 15, 16, 17, **18,** 19, 20, 21, 22, **23,** etc.

Figures in **bold** (3, 8, 13, 18, 23) are those which have been chosen for the sample.

A stratified sample

A stratified sample is obtained by selecting separate random samples from each population stratum. A population can be divided into different groups perhaps

Student	Score (%)	Sample
		TABLE 6.1 STRATIFIED SAMPLING
I	81–100	10% of these students sampled
II	61–80	10% of these students sampled
III	41–60	10% of these students sampled
IV	21–40	10% of these students sampled
V	0–20	10% of these students sampled

based on some characteristic or variable, such as income or education. You can then randomly select from each stratum a given number of units.

In Table 6.1, the exam results range from 0–100%; they are then divided into five strata named I–V.

A cluster sample

As the name implies, a cluster sample is obtained by selecting clusters from a population. Though it may be very economical, cluster sampling can be very susceptible to sampling bias. For example, we may wish to look at discharge times following back surgery in a large city; if we take a cluster of hospitals, we run several risks. Look at Figure 6.3 – it is possible that the cluster all have the same consultant working in them, or the same management team who has set discharge targets, which are not the same as the other hospitals in the city.

Purposeful sampling

Purposeful (purposive) sampling selects information-rich cases for in-depth study. Size and specific cases

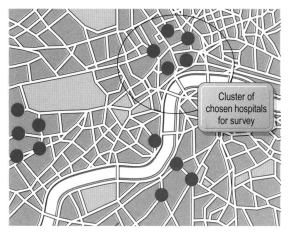

Fig. 6.3 Cluster sampling.

depend on the study purpose. Let us assume that you are doing a qualitative survey into exercise behaviour in cardiac rehabilitation and you know that there are three subgroups of people in whom you are interested:

1. People who exercise every day.
2. People who exercise once a week.
3. People who never exercise.

In this case, you deliberately set out to sample for each of these three groups (Fig. 6.4).

Snowball sampling

You may remember, as a child, you rolled a snowball down a hill and as the snowball rolled it gained more and more snow and by the time you had reached the

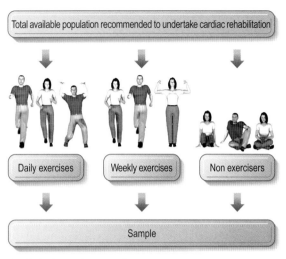

Fig. 6.4 Purposive sampling.

bottom of the hill, you had a large snowball. There is a technique known as snowball sampling which mimics this (Fig. 6.5).

From a single subject, it is possible to quickly build a sample of subjects.

Snowball sampling may be useful when trying to overcome the problems associated with sampling concealed populations, such as those who have sexually transmitted diseases (Kalichman et al. 2000) or substance abuse (Seth et al. 2005).

Snowball sampling can be applied, as an informal method to reach target populations. It is used most frequently when conducting qualitative research, primarily

Person 1 finds people 2,3 and 4 who then each find another
3 people and so on

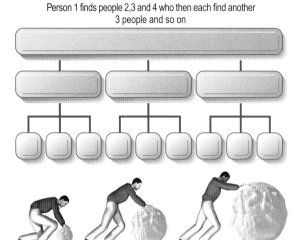

Fig. 6.5 Snowball sampling.

through interviews. Snowball sampling enables the researcher to access populations that may otherwise remain inaccessible. Often, members of such populations may be involved in activities that are considered deviant, such as drug taking or prostitution. Trust is often developed as referrals are made by friends rather than other more formal methods of identification. The required number of links in a referral chain varies depending upon the needs of the study.

VALIDITY

A test or a measure is said to be a valid one when it measures what it is supposed to measure. How valid a test will be depends on its purpose, for example, an X-ray of the spine may be a valid test for measuring the degree of joint wear and tear, but is not valid for measuring the amount of pain that a person experiences. First, we are going to use a simple example here (Fig. 6.6) to explain the concepts of reliability and validity, then we will define the various types of validity that exist.

Types of validity

- *Face validity:* Does the item appear to measure what it is supposed to measure?
- *Content validity:* Is the full content of a concept's definition included in the measure? (Similar to face validity but at a higher level.) The theory behind content validity, as opposed to face validity, is that experts are aware of subtleties in the construct of which the layperson may not be aware.
- *Criterion validity:* Is the item consistent with what we know and expect about a particular topic?
- *Predictive validity:* Predicts a known association between the construct being measured, e.g. me and something else. For example, if someone scores higher on an IQ test, does that predict that they will get a higher degree classification?
- *Concurrent validity:* The validity that is linked with pre-existing indicators, such as something that already measures the same concept, e.g. does your survey on pain give you scores that agree with other things that go along with pain?

Three students are taking an archery class

Example 1 Bill. Every time he fires an arrow it lands in a different place, sometimes he even misses the target completely. There is no reliability (repeatability) to his archery.

Example 2 Andrew. Here Andrew is reliable but not valid, in other words he can be relied upon to repeatedly miss the target in a consistent manner! but does not hit a valid target.

Example 3 Billy. Here Billy is both reliable and valid, he can be relied upon to repeatedly hit the bulls-eye of the archery target. His results are consistent and he does what he sets out to do, i.e. he has reliability and validity.

Fig. 6.6 The concepts of reliability and validity.

- *Construct validity:* Shows that the measure relates to a variety of other measures as specified in a theory. Do the scores that your survey produced correlate with other related constructs in a manner that you could predict?
- *Discriminant validity:* when the measure does not associate with constructs that should not be related.

Validity is an element of social science research which addresses the issues of whether the researcher is actually measuring what they say they are measuring.

Threats to validity

These are factors that can affect how valid a test is:

- *Testing:* A person's past experience of taking a test may have an influence on results. For example if you failed your driving test because you did not know what a particular road sign meant, you are unlikely to make the same mistake the next time you take your driving test.
- *History:* Outside events occurring during the course of the experiment may have an influence on the results, e.g. if a patient changes their medication part way through your research study, it may affect the pain levels that you are researching.
- *Maturation:* Change due to ageing or development. For example, if you do a survey of attitudes of university students in their first week of term, then you should not expect these results to be valid for students at the end of the year.
- *Instrumentation:* The reliability of an instrument may change in calibration (if using a measuring

device) or from change in human error, e.g. if you are measuring the range of movement in a person's knee, different people will measure slightly differently. Even the same person may measure differently if they become fatigued and so on.

- *Selection:* The participants in groups may be unalike in one or more ways.
- *Mortality:* Participants drop out of the test, making the groups unequivalent.
- *Placebo effect:* People may improve due to their hopes and beliefs, rather than the treatment itself.
- *Hawthorne effect:* People's participation in the study makes them feel special – so they act differently, regardless of what is done to them.

RELIABILITY

If you have a car that starts every morning, never lets you down and always gets you to work, it is said to be reliable, in other words, its performance is repeatable.

Reliability has to do with the quality of measurement. In its everyday sense, reliability is the 'consistency' or 'repeatability' of your measures.

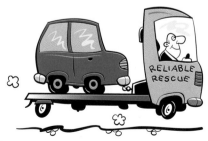

Fig. 6.7

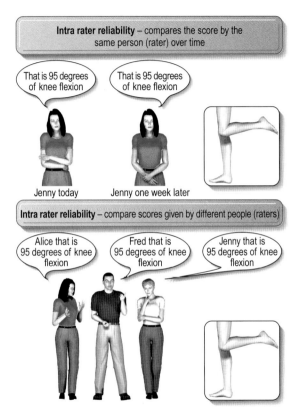

Fig. 6.8   Intra and inter reliability.

It is important to realise that no measurement is perfect, but there are things that you can do to make the data as reliable as possible, there are statistical tests that look at how consistent the questions in a questionnaire are, e.g. Cronbachs Alpha is one useful example if you have set a questionnaire – ask your statistician to explain this to you.

- *Intra rater reliability:* Looks at whether the same person over time makes the same readings of a measure.
- *Inter rater reliability:* Looks at whether different observers are consistent or not.

LEARNING OUTCOMES

After reading this chapter you should have a basic understanding of . . .
- What a sample is
- Why you need to sample
- What types of samples exist
- An overview of reliability and validity.

REFERENCES

Kalichman S C, Rompa D, Cage M 2000 Sexually transmitted infections among HIV seropositive men and women. Sexually Transmitted Infections 76(5):350–354.

Seth R, Kotwal A, Ganguly K K 2005 Street and working children of Delhi, India, misusing toluene: an ethnographic exploration. Substance Use & Misuse 40(11):1659–1679.

CHAPTER SEVEN

Presenting your research and speaking to others

Susan Porter and Stuart Porter

According to most studies, people's number one fear is public speaking. Number two is death. Death is number two! Does that sound right? This means to the average person, if you go to a funeral, you're better off in the casket than doing the eulogy.

(Anonymous)

At some point you will be expected to present your research or some other part of your academic study. This chapter makes things a little easier for you.

GETTING YOUR POINT ACROSS

Truly great speakers can achieve their aims very quickly. On 1 July, 1863, American Union and Confederate **173** forces met in battle at Gettysburg. After the battle, the famous public speaker, Edward Everett, spoke at the dedication at the cemetery. He also invited President Abraham Lincoln. Everett spoke for well over 2 hours, but his speech has long since been forgotten.

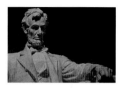

Fig. 7.1 With permission from © Getty images.

Abraham Lincoln then stood and said 237 words – leaving the audience stunned. That speech, know as the 'Gettysburg Address', is now widely accepted as one of the greatest speeches ever written. Here it is:

Four score and seven years ago our fathers brought forth, upon this continent, a new nation, conceived in liberty, and dedicated to the proposition that all men are created equal. Now we are engaged in a great civil war, testing whether that nation, or any nation so conceived, and so dedicated, can long endure. We are met on a great battle field of that war. We have come to dedicate a portion of it, as a final resting place for those who died here, that the nation might live. This we may, in all propriety do. But, in a larger sense, we can not dedicate – we can not consecrate – we can not hallow, this ground – The brave men, living and dead, who struggled here, have hallowed it, far above our poor power to add or detract. The world will little note, nor long remember what we say here; while it can never forget what they did here.

It is rather for us, the living, to stand here, we here be dedicated to the great task remaining before us – that, from these honored dead we take increased devotion to that cause for which they here, gave the last full measure of devotion – that we here highly resolve these dead shall not have died in vain;

that the nation, shall have a new birth of freedom, and that government of the people by the people for the people, shall not perish from the earth.

What makes a presentation good?

There are three things to aim at in public speaking: first, to get into your subject, then to get your subject into yourself, and lastly, to get your subject into the heart of your audience

(Alexander Gregg)

The chances are that you are currently an undergraduate student. Ironically, by now, from your own student experiences, you probably already know better than the experts what makes a good presentation or lecture and what makes a bad one. When you come to do your own, you will adopt your own style but here are some guidelines to help you in the early stages.

> **TIP**   Remember to follow any guidelines that have been supplied to you, failure to follow guidelines really frustrates examiners. Bear in mind that often the presentation of research follows strict protocols and the flexibility that is possible in other lectures, is often not possible.

To avoid the 'opening jitters', practice the opening of your presentation. When you are driving to the location of the presentation, keep saying the first few minutes over and over. You do not have to say it the same each time, just practice the beginning. Your fear of the audience is misplaced, as audiences are usually interested in what you have to say.

TIP Do not start your presentation by apologising and stating that you are nervous, they have probably heard it all before and know that already!

Time your presentation: go through the whole thing *out loud* at least once without interruption. You will then get a realistic idea of how long it will take.

- Concentrate on knowing the content of your presentation
- Also – know your audience – who are they and what is their existing knowledge?

In the case of research presentations, the audience will probably be looking for you to convince them that you have a sound understanding of the research process and a basic understanding of the methods and methodology that you used (we will explain these terms later). Tell the audience at the outset whether they need to make their own notes or not and what handouts will be supplied. This reassures the audience and allows them to relax and concentrate. Pitch your presentation at the right level. This is tricky – do not insult their intelligence, but do not show off either. Think about what they are looking for from your presentation and think about how you can best get the message across.

TIP Be professional but not too slick – this annoys the audience, do not try to be funny unless you are talking about a subject in which you are a world leader – with all respect, this scenario is unlikely at undergraduate level.

THE VENUE

Make sure you know about the room or lecture hall that you will be speaking in.

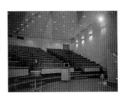

Fig. 7.2

- How big is the room?
- Where will you stand?
- What equipment do you need?
- Provision of a drink if you get a dry mouth?
- Where are the emergency exits?

Tell the audience:

- What you are going to cover
- Why you are covering it
- How you propose to cover it
- . . . and finally, summarise what you told them.

Think of the likely questions that you could be asked and rehearse your answers in front of a friend. There are standard questions that examiners like to ask about research projects and we will cover these later.

If things go wrong, audiences appreciate and are relaxed by presenters who can roll with it. Have back-up technology available: if you are using a laptop, bring a memory stick with the presentation on and/or some paper copies. Cover all eventualities of technology malfunction.

> **TIP** Paper copies do not crash. Your audience will not have any sympathy with you if they have to wait while you find another laptop or compatible software.
> Audiences expect that this will have been checked out previously – even though most people in the audience have committed the same error.

Do not assume someone has arranged for the overhead or slide projector; make a call yourself to make sure.

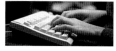

Fig. 7.3

PowerPoint can destroy an audience's will to stay awake. In some respects, Power-Point is actually worse than the old acetates that teachers used to use. PowerPoint is usually accompanied by the monotonous hum of a laptop computer and the endless attempts of the student to add humour, as many words as possible and other bells and whistles to the presentation.

TIP You may need to practise so you can effectively use a remote mouse. A remote mouse is essential so that you do not have to stay glued to the computer.

FACILITATING THE AUDIENCE

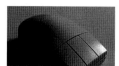

Fig. 7.4

Now you are ready to commence the presentation, so here are a few tips to make the presentation run smoothly:

- Be positive – this will help to create a good atmosphere
- Make the purpose and procedure clear – set an agenda with the audience
- Establish your authority and right to be there
- Create the right atmosphere
- Generate interest and enthusiasm
- Be perceived as professional – even if you do not feel so.

Make it personal

Make eye contact.

Looking at people in your audience for longer than one second is one of the keys of successfully engaging your audience. End your sentences looking at a person, not at the screen. Many presenters end a key point they are making with their eyes on the screen or the laptop and this just

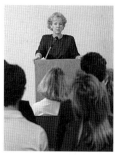

Fig. 7.5

shows your audience you are not interested in them. It may also give the message that you are interested in getting the presentation done as soon as possible.

Pause between points

Most people are too busy. They run from one task to another. When they get up to present they ramble from one point to the next, never allowing a moment of silence in the room. When you are giving a key point in your talk, say it slower, look at people and pause at the end of the point. This will tell your audience that you are saying something that is very important to them. You want them to take a moment to think about it. Never underestimate the power of the pause, it allows your audience to digest what you have said; it can emphasise a particular point you wish the audience to concentrate on and it can also allow you to collate your thoughts before moving onto the next topic.

It's about the story, not the storyteller

Imagine for a moment that we took the story away from the storyteller. Remember Jackanory, a children's programme from the 1970s and 1980s. This consisted of a storyteller with a story to tell, a few pictures and a child's vivid imagination; but those stories were worth listening to. In the same way, presentations desperately need a strong underlying story that is appropriate for the audience. This is equally true of research presentations which otherwise can quickly become monotonous and stale.

A strong opening statement

In the opening moments of a presentation, an audience will make a quick determination whether the presentation they are about to sit through is about them, the presenter or their prowess with software and technology. Use the opening moments of a presentation to set the stage, create clear relevance to an audience and thereby creating empathy enabling you to get the audience on your side. A good start will also help you overcome any initial moments of nervousness.

Well-orchestrated and rehearsed conclusion

Far too often, presentations appear to end not because there is a clear conclusion, but rather it seems the presenter ran out of slides, time, or both. A storyteller works hard so their audiences understand the moral of the story. If the whole point of the story is not clearly understood, a good storyteller would be hard pressed to consider the day a success, yet many presenters fly through the end of their presentations with little regard for a crisp, well-rehearsed conclusion. Spend 30% of your practice time simply working on the opening and closing 5–8 min of your presentation. Pull all the pieces together so the audience understands the main points behind your presentation. If your time is cut short, never compromise the time for your closing comments. Abbreviate the depth of description in the middle of the presentation if necessary, but never the conclusion.

* **Don't** play with change in your pockets – If you are nervous there is a good chance you'll start jingling it, which makes you look both nervous and stupid.

* **Don't** pace – a presentation is much more powerful when we stand still and put all our energy into the presentation. Presentations can become lost when the audience spends their time watching the presenter pace.

✔ **Do** look professional – make the effort to look presentable. People's perceptions of you, rightly or wrongly, can be made in the first moments of meeting you and you *want* to create the right impression. It can be difficult to know what to wear – a suit, smart trousers, nice shoes (although I would advise against 4 inch Jimmy Choo's); generally know who you are presenting to – a group of eminent physicians, wear a suit; your colleagues, smart trousers or skirt will suffice.

✔ **Do** use limited hand movements to draw attention to the slide at an important moment.

* **Avoid** excess jewellery, showing tattoos or body piercing, as it will distract from *your* message.

Remember that the audience is on your side – they *want* to know what you have to say or they would not have made the effort to attend the presentation.

✖ **Do not** read from your slides all the time. By all means refer back to them if you are getting lost in your presentation but constantly referring back to the slides will suggest that you are unfamiliar with the presentation matter.

✖ **Do not** make your slides complicated. Create slides that focus on the points you want people to remember. This may sound silly, but in reality it isn't done very often. Use each slide to drive home *one* point – *bullet* points should reinforce this one point.

✖ **Do not** read word-for-word the content of your slides as this will irritate your audience. Instead, let them read the slides while you embellish their content.

✔ **Do** define all abbreviations, never assume that people will understand. Similarly, make sure *you* know what they mean.

✖ **Do not** take more than 3 min per slide. Work out how long you have to present and divide by three; this will dictate how many slides you will need.

✔ **Do** thank the people who asked you to come, and thank your audience.

✔ **Do** prepare a memorable closing statement; make it an effective motivating summary of the presentation.

✔ **Do** use a consistent style of text and font size throughout.

✔ **Do** try to have a good time – presenting can be Hell or Heaven; it is what *you* make it.

Presentation to groups of peers (classmates)

If you are asked to present to your classmates, then you should take the opportunity to do so, some students do not put too much effort into these, since they may not be assessed but this would be a mistake, the more practice that you can get the better, and you will probably get some useful feedback from your fellow students. It is also useful in that you are usually not constrained by the limits of an exam. If you want to use humour then you can do so – just make sure that you know your subject well enough though, as there is nothing more embarrassing than listening to someone who is trying to make up for a lack of knowledge by being funny. Many years ago, I attended a management course at which there were some extremely competent managers, many of whom were women. The speaker entered the room and within 5 min had made a potentially insulting remark about women as managers, which was meant as a joke but unfortunately following this and for the rest of the week, the speaker was viewed with hostility. Although his knowledge of the subject was good, this was not reflected in his feedback at the end of the course. In other words, the audience had remembered context rather than content.

My own view is that some people are natural presenters and this type of chapter will be of no use to them whatsoever. These people have an instinctive ability to sense the needs of their audience, and much like a talented storyteller, are able to take the audience with them. There are also those for whom it does not come naturally at all and these people tend to need much more structure to their presentations.

Presentation to your lecturers

On the whole, your lecturers will be looking for very specific points. Make sure that you know what the marking schedule or allocation of marks will be for, and work to this. Above all, have a good grasp of the method that you have used and its strengths and weaknesses.

Presentation to patients

You may be asked to speak to a group of patients; this will commonly be when you are on clinical placement. For example, you may be speaking to a group of people with back pain. The rules are more or less the same but you will need to change your language. Patients, on the whole, are not interested in phrases like *methodology* or *outcome measures*. Think of yourself in their position what they want to know, which is what your research has found and what is the relevance/benefits/cost to them. Think about the last time you went to the dentist; you were not interested in the type of filling or drill that the dentist was using, you did subconsciously assume that it had been previously researched, what you did want to know was how long would it take, what would it cost and would it hurt! Try not to show off using unnecessarily long words – remember Abraham Lincoln at the start of this chapter.

HOW TO HANDLE CRITICISM OF YOUR PRESENTATION

You may ask why I have incorporated this section into this chapter if everything that has been written is to ensure that you do a good presentation. The answer is simple – you can please some people some of the time but unfortunately you cannot please all of the people all of the time and through the progression of your career, you will come across certain individuals who will object to:

- Your presentation style
- Your choice of research method
- Your subject matter
- Your conclusions.

This is extremely hard to take when you may have put your heart and soul into the presentation; however you must remember this is *not* personal.

We all present differently; after all, we are all individuals, and as such we all have different views. What one researcher thinks is relevant to your findings another may not; a fact that I have found difficult at times despite my many years in academia. Sometimes it seems that no matter how thorough you have been, someone will find holes in it, however this is the way in which good research becomes better research and whenever possible, you should embrace this although it may seem hard to take at the time.

How can you handle negative feedback on what feels like your life's work? This is never an easy question either to answer or to give any kind of theory as to how to handle it – ask my wife, she bears the brunt of it all!

- Remember it is *not* personal, but rather an attempt at offering advice and support
- Listen to what they are saying – is it negative or just the intonation of their voice you are reacting badly to?

- Never reply in anger – avoid a reflex 'knee jerk' response. Instead, listen to what the criticism is, as it might not be as bad as originally thought. Then, if need be, tell them you will get back to them when you have thought about what they have said – they may have a point!

- Never reply immediately to e-mails criticising your work when submitting it. Save the e-mail and go back when less angry and think about what they are trying to say. If you are starting out on the long road to research, they may have been on that road for some years and can give you the benefit of their wisdom.

FORMATTING YOUR PRESENTATION

No one wants their presentation to be dull, uninteresting or monotonous. Presenters in general want their audience to sit up, pay attention, find the content interesting and above all, learn something from the presentation. How can you make sure that this happens with your presentation? You may not have been born with great presentation skills and the ability to design awe-inspiring presentations but it is a skill which can be acquired over time.

Whenever you get the chance, when sitting in or observing a presentation, pay attention and learn from the presentation you are witnessing.

- Is the screen layout easy to understand?
- Does the colour strengthen or hamper the presentation?
- Is the text easy to read? Are there spelling mistakes or grammatical errors?

- Do the graphics compliment the presentation or are they sending different messages?
- How did the presenters do in their presentation? What did they do well, what could they have done differently?

As you travel through the academic world, you will start to have an idea what makes a great presentation and what makes a really bad one, so when it comes to your turn, you will have a good sound starting base with which to develop your presentation.

How to get started

Start with a plan. Planning the entire presentation: timeframes, equipment, scheduling, etc. helps to identify key elements and progress against time, thereby ensuring that you are fully prepared.

- Planning at every stage helps you to identify any problems and spot them early enough so that you may avoid them
- Planning also helps you to decide upon the resources that you will need along the way and enable you to make provisions for them
- Above all, planning the presentation from an early stage helps to assist your mind to ponder over your message.

Once the background to the presentation has been established, along with the venue, technical equipment, audience, etc., it is time to start the planning of the content and the first stage of this is to plan the structure of the presentation.

- *Title:* The title to your presentation should be clear and succinct to indicate the content of the presentation.
- *Introduction:* The introduction forms the first part of your presentation and lays the groundwork for the entire presentation. The first few minutes of the presentation are vital, as they lay the cornerstone of the entire presentation; therefore it is imperative that you present all the essential aspects of the presentation at this point. The introduction should take no more than a few minutes; any longer and you risk losing your audience.
- *Body:* The body of the presentation is where the substance of your research is presented. This section is also where most of your visual presentation will take place: your findings, facts and figures. Where possible, it is important to make the visual aids as simple as possible, otherwise your audience will spend the majority of their time figuring out what you mean by your slide, rather than focusing on what you are saying.
- *Conclusion:* This is the final aspect to your presentation, and the section which should summarise the important aspects of your presentation. The conclusion should include a summary of the aim of the research, key results, conclusions that are drawn from the findings and their implications.

Typical questions that you might be asked when giving a research presentation

- Why did you choose this particular method?
- What are the strengths and weaknesses of this method?

- Have you thought about using this method instead?
- What do your findings add to the body of knowledge?
- How does your work fit in with the findings of Smith?
- How would you change it next time?
- What are the clinical implications for your work?
- What have you learned on your research journey?

Practice answering these questions before your presentation.

POSTER PRESENTATIONS

With thanks to Ming Tham, Department of Chemical and Process Engineering, University of Newcastle upon Tyne, UK

As part of your degree course or at conventions and meetings it is now common practice to be asked to present a poster presentation. A poster is a visual medium that you use to communicate ideas and messages. The difference between *poster* and *oral* presentations is that you should let your poster do most of the 'talking'; that is, the material presented should convey the essence of your research message. In conferences, you are usually expected to stand-by-your-poster. Your task as the presenter is to answer questions and provide further details; to bask in praises or suffer difficult questions.

How much poster space are you allowed?

The purpose of poster presentations is not to have boards upon boards of information. If you are presenting your poster at a conference or convention, you will have limited space. Find out how much space you are allowed before you commence planning the project, since the space you are allowed will determine the content of the poster.

Is there a standard format?

As with an oral presentation, there is normally a:

- *Title page:* telling others the title of the project, the people involved in the work and their affiliation
- *Summary* of the project stating what you have set out to do, how you have done it, the key findings and the main results
- *Introduction* which should include clear statements about the problem or question that you are trying to address. These should then lead to your aims and objectives
- *Methodology section:* this explains the basis of the technique that you are using or the procedure that you have adopted in your study. You should also state and justify any assumptions, so that your results could be viewed in the proper context
- *Results section* which you use to show illustrative examples of the main results of the work
- *Conclusion,* listing the main findings of your investigation
- *Further work section* that should contain your recommendations and thoughts about how the

work could be progressed; other tests that could be applied, etc.

You therefore have to present certain pieces of information but with limited space. Unlike oral presentations, where some ultra-smooth talkers may be able to divert attention from a poorly planned presentation, with posters, poor planning is there for all to see.

Gathering the information

First, ask yourself the following questions:

- What is the objective of the research?
- Has someone previously done this work or similar work?
- How have I approached my study?
- Why did I follow this particular route of investigation?
- What are the principles governing the technique that I am using?
- What assumptions did I make and what are my justifications?
- What problems did I encounter?
- What results did I obtain?
- Have I solved the problem?
- What have I found out?
- Are the analyses sound?

You have to stand back and think again about the *Whats*, the *Hows* and the *Whys* of the work that you have done. You have to examine critically, the approach that you have taken and the results that you have. Be ruthless in your assessment of yourself – better to be a masochist than the victim of a sadist.

Ideally, you should have done this throughout your project anyway. In doing so, you will have a clearer idea of the objectives and the contributions that you have, or have not, been able to make. This means that you will know better, the information you have at your disposal for presentation.

Deciding on the content

You now have to decide between what is important and what is not necessary. Your decision should be based on at least two factors:

What are you trying to achieve by presenting the poster?

■ Is it to tell people what you have done? Is it to tell people of a new discovery? Is it to convince people that one product or technique is better than another?

Who will be attending the presentation?

■ What is the level of their knowledge of your subject area and what are they likely to be looking for?

The answers to these questions define the *type of content* to include and set the *tone of the presentation*.

Keep the material simple

- Make full use of the space, but do not cramp a page full of information, as the result can often appear messy
- Be concise and do not waffle. Use only pertinent information to convey your message
- Be selective when showing results. Present only those that illustrate the main findings of the project. However, do keep other results handy so that you may refer to them if/when asked.

Use colours sparingly

- Colours should be used only to emphasise and differentiate. Do not use colours just to impress
- Try to avoid using large swathes of bright garish colours like bright green, pink, orange or lilac
- Pastel shades convey feelings of serenity and calm, while heavy bright colours conjure images of conflict
- Choose background and foreground colour combinations that have high contrast and complement each other – black or dark blue on white or very light grey is good
- It is better to keep the background light as people are used to it (e.g. in newspapers and books)
- Avoid the use of gradient fills. They may look great on a computer display, but unless you have access to a high-resolution printer, the paper version can look tatty.

Do not use more than two font types

- *Titles* and *headings* should appear larger than other text, but not too large. The text should also be legible from a distance, say from 1.5 m to 2 m.
- *Do not use all UPPER CASE type in your posters.* It can make the material difficult to read. Just compare the two sentences below:

WHAT DO YOU THINK OF THIS LINE WHERE ALL THE CHARACTERS ARE IN UPPER CASE?

What do you think of this line, where only the first character of the first word is in upper case?

Do not use a different font type to highlight important points

- Otherwise the fluency and flow of your sentence can appear disrupted
- Use <u>underlined text</u>, the **bold face** or *italics* or ***combinations*** to emphasise words and phrases
- If you use ***bold italicised print*** for emphasis, then <u>***underlining***</u> is not necessary – overkill!

A picture is worth a thousand words . . . (but only if it is drawn properly and used appropriately)

- Graphs
  - choose graph types that are appropriate to the information that you want to display
  - annotations should be large enough, and the lines of line-graphs should be thick enough so that they may be viewed from a distance

- – do not attempt to have more than six line-graphs on a single plot
- – instead of using lines of different thickness, use contrasting coloured lines or *different line styles* to distinguish between different lines in multi-line graphs
- – multi-line plots or plots with more than one variable should have a legend relating the plotted variable to the colour or style of the line.
- ■ Diagrams and drawings
  - – should be labelled
  - – drawings and labels should be large and clear enough so that they are still legible from a distance
  - – do not try to cramp labelling to fit into components of a drawing or diagram. Use 'arrows' and 'callouts'.
- ■ ClipArt
  - – should only be used if they add interest to the display *and* complement the subject matter. Otherwise, all they do is to distract attention from the focus of the presentation
  - – can also be 'dangerous' as you may spend more time fiddling about with images and choosing appropriate cartoons than concentrating on the content.

Check your spelling

- ■ Spelling mistakes give the impression that you have not put in the effort; careless; not bothered; not worthy of high assessment scores.

Maintain a consistent style

- Inconsistent style gives the impression of disharmony and can interrupt the fluency and flow of your messages
- Headings on the different pages of the poster should appear in the same position on all pages
- Graphs should be of the same size and scale, especially if they are to be compared
- If bold lettering is used for emphasis on one page, then do not use italics on others
- Captions for graphs, drawings and tables should either be positioned at the top or at the bottom of the figure.

The arrangement of poster components should appear smooth

- You would probably prepare sections of the poster on A4-sized paper before sticking them onto mounting boards or display stands
- Remember that you are using posters to tell a story about what you have done and achieved. As in report writing, the way you arrange the sections should follow the 'storyline'
- Sometimes it is helpful if you provide cutouts of arrows to direct attention to the sequence of the presentation
- Use a new page to start off a new section.

Review, review and review

Make draft versions of your poster sections and check them for:

- ■ Mistakes
- ■ Legibility and
- ■ Inconsistency in style.

Ask your partner, friends, colleagues or supervisor for their honest opinions – be critical yourself.

 USEFUL WEB LINK Dr Ming Tham maintains a web page with useful information about presentations: http://lorien.ncl.ac.uk/ming/Dept/Tips/present/present.ht

Figure 7.6 is a suggested layout for a poster.

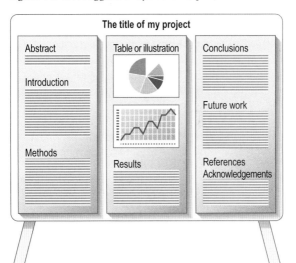

Fig. 7.6

WHAT EXAMINERS LOOK FOR . . .

We will now compare the people that are going to examine and mark your research, to sharks, no insult is intended but I think that this will be a useful analogy.

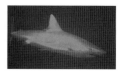

Fig. 7.7

Imagine that you are swimming among a shoal of sharks. The sharks are docile and happy to swim around you, occasionally nudging you if you are in their way; other than that, no harm comes to you, the sharks are interested in you, but you have a nice time as long as you behave.

Now let us assume that you swim the next day but you carelessly cut your leg and it starts to bleed. This arouses the shark's interest. As they sense a weakness, they start to swarm around you and begin approaching from all directions; this makes you splash around a lot which arouses the sharks appetite and . . . You can work out the rest!

Do not give the examiner any reason to find obvious mistakes in your research (this equals drops of blood in the water). If you submit a thesis or research protocol which is watertight, i.e. it follows the guidelines, is well presented and has no grammatical or typographical errors, then you might say that the examiners are more likely to behave like the docile sharks, academically speaking they will nudge you but there will be no blood.

Now consider the situation of the student who submits a piece of work which has coffee stains on the front cover; the work has no page numbers; no acknowledgements section and the references in the reference list do not match those cited in the text. To make matters worse, a spell check has not been done and it appears that many of the guidelines that were stressed so meticulously 6 months previously, have been ignored. In academic terms, this student is bleeding profusely and arousing the interest of the sharks to the point where they may undertake a feeding frenzy – i.e. they will pick apart your work and virtually destroy it, before the reader even gets down to studying the actual content. They are also far less likely to let the odd minor error go, than if the rest of the work had been of high quality.

Here are some of the common mistakes that examiners frequently pick up on:

- Spelling mistakes on both medical and non-medical words
- The work fails to clearly state the aim or research question
- The work is descriptive with no depth of analysis
- No page numbers
- No labels on illustrations
- The work fails to follow a consistent thread after stating the aim or research question
- Sentences that do not make sense
- References cited that do not match those in the reference list
- Generally hard work to read.

Time and again lecturers and examiners supply detailed guidelines and time and again they know that a proportion of students will not adhere to them. Do not feed the sharks!

TIPS ON USING POWERPOINT

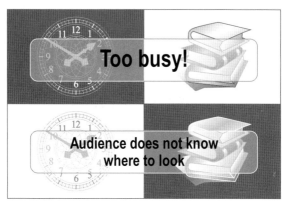

Fig. 7.8

THIS ONE USES ALL
CAPITALS, IT IS HARD TO
READ AND LOOKS AS
THOUGH YOU ARE SHOUTING!

Fig. 7.9

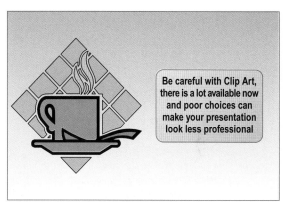

Fig. 7.10

Some students simply put too much information on each slide and as a result they have to wait while the audience reads through the text and simultaneously lose the will to live.

Most people will not bother to read the entire text, this is a shame since you probably have some key facts and important information contained within the text.

Also don't make the text too small, this adds effort to the job of the audience. Make sure that you stick to bullet points that are relevant, do not digress and start talking about non-essential information.

Fig. 7.11

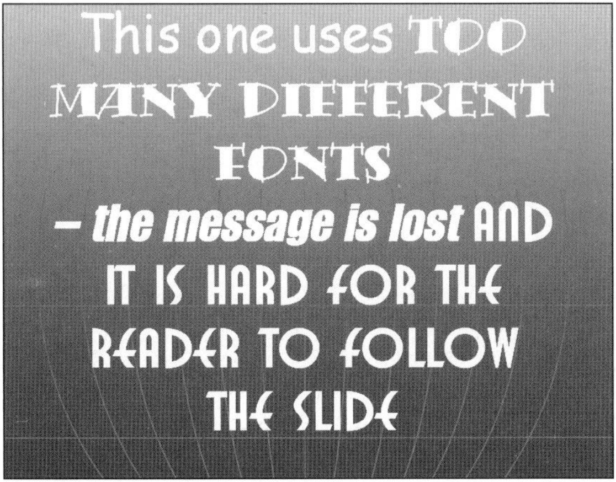

Fig. 7.12

LEARNING OUTCOMES

After reading this chapter you should have a basic understanding of . . .

- How to get your point across
- What makes a presentation good
- How to handle criticism
- How to format your presentation
- Typical questions you will be asked
- How to succeed in poster presentations
- Suggested layout for a poster
- What examiners look for – sharks in the water
- Using PowerPoint.

CHAPTER EIGHT

Carrying out qualitative research

Maggie Donovan-Hall and Bridget Dibb

So when you are listening to somebody, completely, attentively, then you are listening not only with words, but also to the feeling of what is being conveyed, to the whole of it, not part of it

(Jiddu Krishnamuri, Indian Theosophist Philosopher, 1895–1986)

This chapter aims to introduce the novice researcher to qualitative research. 'Qualitative research' is an umbrella term for different methodologies and approaches; however, it is not possible to provide an extensive overview all of these approaches in just one chapter. This chapter will therefore concentrate on the aims of qualitative data collection and analysis mainly used in undergraduate research. References and Further

Reading will be provided to guide you to sources of additional qualitative methods.

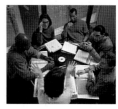

Fig. 8.1

THE AIM OF QUALITATIVE RESEARCH

As noted in Chapter 2, quantitative research is embedded within the positivist (or scientific) paradigm and is based on the assumption that there is one objective truth that can be sought by objectively measuring and analysing data. In contrast to the positivist approach, qualitative research is not concerned with trying to measure a single objective truth, but proposes that there are many different truths relating to the individual's subjective and cultural experiences (Murray & Chamberlain 1998). Indeed, as noted by Finlay & Ballinger (2006:6), 'Qualitative research aims to investigate and understand the social world rather than predict, explain and control behaviour'. Unlike quantitative research, which involves quantification of all variables, qualitative research acknowledges that not all things can be expressed numerically and some things need to be studied in depth and in detail. Therefore, the aim of qualitative research is to attempt to capture the participants' perceptions, thoughts and experiences, which will provide an holistic overview of the issue that is being investigated (Fig. 8.1).

It is worth clarifying that despite being fundamentally different, both qualitative and quantitative approaches are valuable methods of inquiry. Gone are the days where quantitative methods took precedence and qualitative research was viewed as the 'poor relation' (Barbour 2003:1019) battling for inclusion in mainstream journals. Indeed, over the last 50 years, qualitative research has gained increasing power and respect. It is now more widely recognised that both qualitative and quantitative approaches employ methods that are rigorous, systematic and logical (Mays & Pope 1995).

Furthermore, as the qualitative researcher is interested in understanding the individual's social experiences, it acknowledges that information gathered will reflect the individual's subjective social experiences and therefore it does not aim to produce findings that can be generalised to the wider population (i.e. it does not aim to find a fixed truth). Compared with quantitative research that aims to present representative samples of participants, qualitative research normally involves recruiting smaller groups of participants.

As qualitative research is interested in exploring how people make sense of the world and their social experiences, it is also understood that these issues are subject

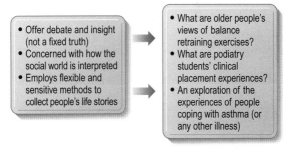

Fig. 8.2 A summary of the aim of qualitative research and possible questions.

to interpretation and it is likely that other researchers' interpretations of the same data would present different findings. However, as noted in Chapter 2, unlike quantitative research, which aims to make a clear separation between the researcher and participant, within qualitative research it is accepted that 'the researcher is a central figure who influences, and perhaps actively constructs, the collection, selection and interpretation of data' (Finlay & Ballinger 2006:6).

WHAT IS MY RESEARCH QUESTION?

Having taught research methods to undergraduate allied healthcare students for several years, it has become apparent that 'some' students decide to carry out a qualitative research project purely because they hate the thought of doing statistics.

First, we want to reassure you that the statistics monster does not really exist and you should not be scared of statistics (even if you do still believe in the statistics monster, it can be slain with hard work and determination). Second, we would like to reinforce the point made in Chapter 1, which stated that your research question should dictate the method you select and not the other way around. Qualitative research aims to explore people's experiences, perceptions and views and does not test the relationships between variables. For example, if you are interested in determining whether there is a relationship between fear of falling and physical exercise levels in older people, this will involve quantitative research methods. This could be done by using standardised questionnaires to provide numerical representation of the level of fear of falling and the physical activity and statistical analysis could be used

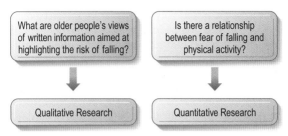

Fig. 8.3 Does your research question reflect qualitative or quantitative methods?

to explore relationships between these two variables. Alternatively, if you were interested in exploring older people's views on written information of the risk of falling, this question would be best addressed through asking older people their thoughts, feelings and experiences about falls prevention advice and would therefore involve qualitative research methods.

HOW SHALL I COLLECT MY QUALITATIVE DATA?

As the aim of qualitative research is to gain an understanding of how people's experiences are shaped by their social experiences and social-cultural backgrounds, ways of collecting this information may be in the form of the spoken or written word (e.g. individuals reflecting on their life experiences or writing diaries), or the actual observation of behaviour (Seale & Barnard 1998). Indeed, there are many different ways to collect qualitative data, such as interviews, focus groups, action research, observations and carrying out a case study approach. However, within qualitative research, interviews and focus groups have been reported as the most widely used means of obtaining qualitative data. Maybe the ability to organise these methods of data collection within the right time frames of most research projects contributes to their popularity in undergraduate research. Therefore, this chapter will only focus on these two techniques and will aim to provide a brief overview of the advantages and disadvantages of each technique, followed by systematic guidelines for you to follow.

Carrying out interviews

When carrying out an enquiry involving humans, why not take advantage of the fact that they can tell you things about themselves

(Robson 1997:227)

Interviews provide the opportunity for you to explore your research question and directly ask participants about their specific inner thoughts and feelings. However, in order to obtain rich and insightful data, it is important that your interviews are carefully planned and you try to learn some good interview techniques.

Types of interviews

Interviews are normally carried out face-to-face or on the telephone. Telephone interviews are often regarded as a cheaper and quicker method of interviewing, as they save time and money on travelling to the interview and therefore, can widen the geographical area of participant recruitment. However, it may be found that the relationship between the interviewer and participant is restrained and it is difficult to gauge the participant's

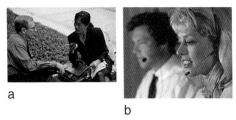

a

b

Fig. 8.4 Choosing the right tool for the right job is very important in qualitative research. (a) Face-to-face and (b) telephone interviews.

reactions to certain questions. Face-to-face interviews therefore provide a better opportunity for the interviewer to observe any non-verbal information that may aid the understanding of the verbal responses.

In addition to the way that the interviews are carried out, there are several different types of interview formats. The type of format you wish to employ will relate to your interview schedule and they are generally categorised as structured, semi-structured and unstructured (depth) interviews.

Structured interviews

Structured interviews involve a structured interview schedule containing a set of fixed (closed-ended) questions that are read out in an identical manner to each participant. These questions are often accompanied by a set of fixed answers and the participant selects the most appropriate answer to match their view. These fixed responses are normally provided with a numerical code and therefore provide quantitative data. Although structured interviews with set answers are essentially the same as a spoken questionnaire, delivery in an interview format provides the researcher with the opportunity to clarify any questions that the participant may not understand and ensure that all of the questions are answered (Drummond 1996). Although open-questions are often included at the end of the interview schedule, where the participant is free to say what they want (e.g. Do you have anything else to add about . . .?), this type of interview normally obtains short factual answers (Seale & Barnard 1998). As this method does not provide the participant with the opportunity to discuss their experiences and views in depth, it is not generally employed within qualitative studies that aim to collect rich information (Wilkinson et al. 2004).

Semi-structured interviews
Unlike the structured interview that aims to obtain factual information, the semi-structured interview involves a set of broad open-ended questions that the interviewer is free to modify. In order to obtain the participant's own beliefs and perceptions about the subject matter, the questions need to be carefully worded in an open and non-directive manner. Such modifications may involve changing the wording and order of the questions, including additional prompts to further explore the participant's response, and missing out later questions if they have already been answered or seem inappropriate based on the participant's responses to earlier questions. These types of interviews are viewed as being particularly useful for exploring complex issues and can provide a detailed picture of the participant's experiences.

Table 8.1 provides an outline of some of the stages that are normally involved in developing a semi-structured interview schedule.

TABLE 8.1	DEVELOPING A SEMI-STRUCTURED INTERVIEW SCHEDULE
Stage 1:	Clearly define your research question.
Stage 2:	Identify broad topics that explore this research question (use your literature review as a guide).
Stage 3:	Use these topics to construct open-ended questions (remember that these questions will only act as a guideline and can be modified).
Stage 4:	Put these questions into a logical order, starting with some easier questions and leaving the more sensitive topics to the end. Make sure that you use: Neutral rather than leading questions Open rather than closed questions Avoid double-barrelled questions (i.e. two questions in one) Avoid using jargon and keep language simple Ask questions that are likely to elicit events and personal questions.
Stage 5:	Add some introductory comments. Make sure that you: Introduce the participant to the topic area Explain who you are and what questions you will be asking A good clear introduction will help relax the participant and therefore it is important that you try to act naturally and do not read straight from a script.

Continued

TABLE 8.1   DEVELOPING A SEMI-STRUCTURED INTERVIEW SCHEDULE *cont.*

Stage 6:	Add some closing comments. This is your opportunity to debrief your participants and ensure that taking part in the interview was a good experience for them. This normally involves answering any questions they may have and offering them any information about the subject matter. Do not forget to thank your participants and offer them a summary of the final report.
Stage 7:	Once you have developed your first draft of your interview schedule, it is important that you pilot your interview schedule (e.g. carrying out a practice interview). Piloting your interview schedule will provide you with the opportunity to check the structure of your questions and practice your interview skills. When carrying out your pilot interview, think about what makes a good interviewer, for example: Being a good listener and not talking over the participant Keeping eye contact and showing that you are interested in what your participant has to say Encouraging the participant to present their own viewpoint without making them feel that you are judging them or looking for socially acceptable explanations Taking time and not rushing the interviews It is normally recommended that you tape-record and transcribe your pilot interview(s).
Stage 8:	Following the pilot study, make the final stages to the interview schedule.

Unstructured (depth) interviews

Unlike the semi-structured interview, carrying out an unstructured interview does not involve following a predetermined set of topics or questions and the development of an interview schedule. Alternatively, it is the aim to cover one or two main areas in greater detail and this therefore allows the participant to discuss the issues that are important to them and not just answer the researcher's questions (Seale & Barnard 1998; Wilkinson et al. 2004). As this type of interview does not involve following a set of questions, it is often found that each interview carried out is very different, and for the novice researcher this can make it very difficult to analyse. Furthermore, as this type of interview is more inclined to allow the participant the freedom to direct and choose the topics discussed, it often takes a skilled researcher to ensure that the discussions are still relevant to the research question (Seale & Barnard 1998). For these reasons, it is found that semi-structured interviews are most widely used within undergraduate qualitative projects.

Focus groups

Unlike interviews that are normally carried out on a one-to-one level and involve exploring one person's views of the research topic, focus groups involve drawing together a small group (normally between six to eight participants) to take part in a group discussion relating to

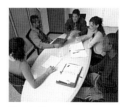

Fig. 8.5

the research question. As with the semi-structured interview, the researcher will have a set of predetermined topics or questions that will be presented to the group (the guidelines in Table 8.1 can be used to develop a focus group schedule). However, instead of asking the questions on an individual level, the researcher normally acts as a moderator and presents the topics to the group and allows natural discussion to take place. As the aim of the focus group is to create naturalistic conversation, the discussion may therefore involve the participants sharing their ideas and experiences or taking part in some debate and possible disagreement. Focus groups also provide you with the opportunity to observe the group dynamics and witness how the discussions are initiated and developed (Wilkinson et al. 2004).

Although focus groups provide the opportunity to explore several people's experiences at one time point, you need to carefully consider whether this is the best methodological approach for your specific research question. It has been noted that as focus groups involve a group discussion, they should not be employed when you intend to ask sensitive questions or if discussions are likely to lead into sensitive areas of discussion. It is also important to consider issues of confidentiality in terms of the group dynamics (e.g. is it likely that the participants will know each other?) and whether you feel that there is any risk that sensitive information may not remain confidential (Krueger & Casey 2000).

If you decide that your research question is suitable for a focus group approach, there are several things that you need to think about at the planning stage of your research.

How many participants in each focus group?

As previously stated, most focus groups generally involve six to eight participants, but can work equally as well with as little as four or as many as ten participants. However, it is important to note that too few participants can restrict the discussion and make people feel pressured, but too many can make it harder to control. With a large focus group, you also run the risk of the participants breaking into smaller discussion groups and not listening to what else is being said. This can obviously have a huge impact on the group dynamics and makes the focus group also impossible to clearly tape-record and transcribe.

How many focus groups will I need to run?

The number of focus groups you are able to run will depend on several factors, such as the availability of your participants, time constraints and your available resources. If you are expecting to invite a very specific sample of individuals that are going to be hard to recruit, this is likely to dictate how many focus groups you are able to run. You also need to think about the amount of time you will have as it will take longer than you think to plan the focus group, recruit the participants and transcribe the data. Because of the number of people within the group and because it is often hard to identify who is talking, transcribing focus group data is considerably harder than transcribing interview data.

Where will I hold the focus group?

The venue where you carry out the focus group is important, as it needs to be a 'neutral' environment for the participants to avoid the participants providing biased and socially acceptable responses. For example, if you want to explore patients' views of physiotherapy, running a focus group within the physiotherapy department may elicit only positive responses. As you will be planning to tape-record the focus group, it is important that you check the noise levels for recording purposes. Most focus groups involve the participants sitting in a circle or around a table with the tape recorder and microphone placed in the middle.

The role of the moderator

In most research, it is normal practice for the researcher to act as the *moderator* (sometimes referred to as the *facilitator*) for the focus group. The role of the moderator is to introduce the topics or questions and encourage on-going discussion by prompting and asking appropriate follow-up questions (Wilkinson et al. 2004). The moderator also needs to ensure that the discussion is focussed on the topic of interest and does not completely digress and provide irrelevant information. This will involve making decisions on whether certain issues raised by the participants should be explored further or skilfully avoided. It is also important that everyone within the focus group is involved in the discussion and it is not just dominated by one or two individuals. From these descriptions, you will see that the moderator's role is not an easy task and therefore you are encouraged to carry out pilot interviews and practice these skills.

The role of the observer

When planning your focus group data collection, it is advised that in addition to your role as the moderator, you get a second person involved to help you run the group. For undergraduate research, this may involve pairing up with another student who is also carrying out focus group research and taking turns helping each other run the groups. This second pair of hands is often referred to as an *observer*, who will be able to make notes on the group dynamics and the non-verbal communication observed. To help with the transcription of the focus group, it is often helpful for the observer to list the order in which the participants talk (e.g. noting the participant's initials and the first couple of words or keywords in the sentence). In addition to observing the focus group and writing notes, the observer often helps with greeting participants on arrival; ensuring that all participants complete a consent form (this should be done at the start of the focus group session); bringing participants refreshments; and checking the recording equipment is working properly.

Running the focus group session

It is important to start the focus group with a good introduction, as this is a good way of relaxing participants and setting the scene of the discussion. The first part of the introduction normally starts with welcoming and thanking participants for taking part; providing an explanation of the study (participants should have already received a Participant Information Sheet and therefore this should be just a brief reminder) and answering any questions they may have. You may then wish to move on to introducing any other members of the focus group team (e.g. the observer) and asking participants to introduce themselves. At this point, it is helpful if the observer makes a note of the seating plan so that they will be aware of who is talking when they list the order of discussion. Before beginning the discussion, it is also recommended that you set some ground rules. This normally involves reminding participants that everything that is said within the focus group should be kept completely confidential and asking them not to talk over each other and respect everyone's opinions.

During the focus group, you need to try to keep the atmosphere as relaxed as possible and do not worry if the focus group takes time to get started (Wilkinson et al. 2004). As a moderator, it is important that you do not try to follow the focus group schedule too rigidly and the discussions should be allowed to flow naturally. As with a semi-structured interview schedule, it is important to start with simple and non-threatening questions, leaving the complex or slightly sensitive questions towards the end.

With regard to drawing the focus group to an end, this may occur naturally once all of the topics of discussion have been addressed and the participants do not have anything else to say. Alternatively, as you would have had to specify how long the focus group will last for on the Participant Information Sheet and your consent form, you may find that you just run out of time and therefore need to bring discussions to a close. Ending the session normally involves asking the participants if they have any further points to add, reassuring issues of confidentiality and thanking the participants (see Wilkinson et al. (2004) for a detailed summary of the focus group process).

How will I get people involved in my research?

Chapter 6 provides a general overview on how to recruit participants to take part in your research. For qualitative research, the general methods used are convenience sampling, purposive sampling and snowballing. However, due to the time restraints of undergraduate research, the majority of projects generally involve recruiting a convenience (or opportunity) sample of participants. Although it will depend on the specific sample of people required, most undergraduate samples are normally recruited through posters being displayed around the university, sending out e-mails and attending local support groups.

HOW WILL I MAKE SENSE OF MY DATA?

After completion of the interviews or focus groups, you need to transcribe the tapes, which is an interesting but quite a time-consuming process. This method allows a full understanding of what the person was saying within the context in which it was said. Once you have transcribed your data, you are ready to begin the analysis. The first stage in this process is the coding stage. You will also need to completely familiarise yourself with the transcripts and this means reading and re-reading until you feel you understand the individual's point of view when they were talking to you at the time of the interview or focus group. The next step involves coding the data and grouping the codes into themes. There are several different ways in which to analyse your data, e.g. interpretative phenomenological analysis, thematic analysis and content analysis to mention three, however, in this chapter we will only be discussing content and thematic analysis as these are the two most common types. At this point, the type of analysis you are using determines which path you take and it is divided into separate sections for content and thematic analysis. Common to both types of analysis is the page layout with which you start your analysis – it is a good idea to widen the margins on the page so that there are large spaces on either side of the text; this allows you the space to write the themes where they arise within the text. At this stage, you should also ensure you have used your computer to number each line on the page. This is important as when you take quotes from the text to insert into the write-up of your research, you are then able to list the line and participant number.

Content analysis

Content analysis involves coding the data according to the determined 'unit of coding'. This can be a word, a phrase, a sentence or a paragraph. Once you have coded, you can add up these codes to determine: (1) what percentage of the participants mentioned that code, and (2) which participant mentioned the code more often. For example, let us say that you wanted to determine whether your participants felt anxious about walking after they had already experienced a fall. You would code the transcripts by highlighting all words or sentences which you interpret as indicating anxiety, e.g. 'I felt nervous . . .', 'I did not feel comfortable when . . .'. These sentences would all be given a code which you could describe as the 'anxious' code, which could then be added up. Should every participant have mentioned a sentence which you coded as showing anxiety you

TABLE 8.2 THEMES EMERGING FROM CONTENT ANALYSIS

Themes	Number of participants	
	n	(%)
Anxiety	10	100
Perceived control	7	70
Social support	3	30
Personal growth	3	30

could conclude that all (100%) of your sample felt anxious with regard to walking after experiencing a fall. You would also be able to discuss how those who had experienced a more recent fall felt more anxious, as they made more anxious comments than those who had experienced a fall some time ago. Results of content analysis are usually presented in a table showing the number of participants for whom the code was important. A sample table (Table 8.2) shows themes emerging from content analysis.

Thematic analysis

While content analysis is concerned with the frequency of the themes, thematic analysis allows the researcher to determine themes which lie within the data; it explores the meaning which the person is trying to convey with their narrative. It is not important how many times a person may refer to that theme, rather, the fact that the theme was mentioned at all is what is

important. To continue with the falls example, should
your participant have mentioned that they feel uncom-
fortable, or worried about walking, you would begin by
writing your initial interpretation of the sort of sentence
or message within the sentence or paragraph (unit of
coding) on the left-hand side of the page. Once you
have done this through the entire transcript, you need
to read through a second time, this time grouping the
theme into an overarching theme within which you feel
the initial theme you coded fits into. It is a good idea
to write this overarching theme on the right-hand side
of the page in order to distinguish it from the lower-
order themes. It is now a good idea to use the participant's own words to describe the theme. For example,
if on reading through the transcript the first time you
had written words such as 'concern', 'worry' or 'anxious',
on the left-hand side of the page, you may, on the
second reading describe all these sub-themes as belong-
ing to the theme of 'anxiousness', which you would
write on the right-hand side of the page. As you read
through subsequent transcripts, you need to follow the
same procedure, allowing for any new, and as yet undis-
covered, themes to be identified as they emerge. The
end result of thematic analysis is a set of themes and
sub-themes which answer the research question. For
example, if you were interested in what factors were
important to people when regaining levels of activity
after a fall, you might find such themes as perception
of control (or lack of), social support, anxiety and personal growth emerging. Your results tell you more about
what is important for this group of people and allow
an indication of factors which may be important for
rehabilitation and adherence to rehabilitation. You

have not determined predictors as that is not what qualitative analysis is about, but you have shown what factors are indicative of the processes at play.

HOW DO I MAKE SURE THAT MY FINDINGS ARE RIGOROUS?

A criticism which qualitative research often faces is that of validity and reliability. Quantitative critics have claimed that as there is no objective standard used in qualitative research and as the data collected are subjective, they are neither valid nor reliable. However, despite the subjective nature of the data in qualitative methods, rigorous and scientific procedures can be followed to ensure that the data are as reliable and valid as possible. In fact, in order to determine how a person feels about an experience, one could argue that the only reliable and valid way to find out is to ask them. Below we discuss steps you can take to ensure your methods are rigorous.

Paper trails

Paper trails refer to the paper evidence of the thoughts and decisions made throughout the study. These include the initial thoughts regarding the conception of the study and subsequent decisions, which need to be well documented. In addition, the recorded tapes of the interviews or focus groups, the transcripts, including the manual coding and theme development, will provide a chain of evidence which can be reviewed by others. This is a way of being transparent about your decisions and it allows others to view how decisions about the study were made and enables them to follow the logical flow of the research process.

Triangulation

Following a robust qualitative method can also involve using 'triangulation'. This is where various different methods may be used to assess the same research question. Using different methods to reach the same result confirms the results, as it shows that the results reached were not influenced by the method. For example, interviews can be used, as well as observation techniques and diaries to collect data from the same group of people. If a theme that emerged from an interview is also present in the diary and observed at, e.g. a support group meeting, we would be justified in choosing this theme. Although there is usually only time to undertake one method in undergraduate research, it is important to be aware of the principle of triangulation for future research and when critically evaluating publications in the literature.

Consult the experts

Experts in the field can be used to verify interview and focus group schedules. A researcher may draw up a list of questions they would like to cover in the interview, all based on what they have read about in the literature and from their own personal experiences. The problem is that there may be other areas not covered in the literature and not experienced by the researcher, which would be omitted from the interview schedule. This may lead to the omission of relevant questions, which in turn means that important answers are not heard. A way to help ensure that as many issues and aspects about the topic as possible have been thought about and included in the schedule is to ask one or two experts to review the schedule and comment on the content.

These comments should be kept as evidence for your paper trail.

Consult the participants

Another method of checking the validity of the data collected is to ask the participants to check and comment on a summary of the discussion. There can be problems associated with this method as, while participants may feel comfortable agreeing with you that you have interpreted their comments accurately, they may view the interviewer as superior to themselves and may therefore be less inclined to disagree with you if they feel you have misinterpreted their comments.

Data saturation

Due to the subjective nature of the data, another criticism may focus on the breadth of the data collected. How can we know that we have every different view on the topic? One way of achieving this is to collect enough data to reach 'data saturation'. When you start to interview, you will find lots of themes emerging from the transcripts, some common to several participants and some different. However, after you have completed several interviews you may find that no new themes emerge from the data of the later interviews. This means you have reached data saturation, i.e. you have collected data reflecting the majority of the themes associated with that topic. This also explains why sample size is not such an issue in qualitative research; the emphasis is on quality, not quantity.

Reflexivity

This concept refers to the awareness a qualitative researcher should have over the impact that they, themselves, may have on the data collection and analysis. Researchers should be aware that the simple act of the interview (or focus group) may create in the participant a different way of thinking about the topic you are asking them about. Just simply asking a participant to think about an issue in a different way may result in a different answer, as you have made them think about it differently. The presence of the interviewer, the way they are dressed, their age, their gender and so on, also have an impact on how the participant views the relationship with the researcher and influences how they respond to questions and the type of answers they may give. Should the participant see you as the 'expert', they may give different answers, perhaps less detail if they think you already know about it. In this way, you can see how the researcher's presence may bias the results. However, reflexivity influences the analysis as well. It is the researcher who reads the transcripts and codes the responses. This same researcher will have experiences, views and preconceived ideas, which will influence their interpretation of the data. The researcher must always be aware that the codes and themes they present are very much 'their' interpretation of the experiences of that group of participants. The researcher should also consider how their interpretation may be influenced by their own experiences and how their interpretations may be different to another researcher.

Inter-rater reliability

Inter-rater reliability is used mainly with content analysis and refers to a method of determining how reliably the researcher has coded the transcripts. It requires another researcher, an independent researcher, to code one of the transcripts. A calculation can then be performed to see how similar the two researchers coded that transcript. The number of agreements is divided by the total number of possible agreements (number of agreements plus number of disagreements). In this way, the level of agreement between the two researchers is determined, a high level of agreement would indicate higher reliability.

Level of agreement = number of agreements ÷ (number of agreements + number of disagreements)

PRESENTATION OF DATA

When you write up qualitative data (both content and thematic analysis), you may combine your analysis section with your discussion, although this can also be done separately. The presentation of the results of a qualitative study should also contribute to providing evidence of the validity of the results. This is done by the presentation of the emerging themes and examples from the data of these themes in the form of quotes. The reader is then in the position to agree or disagree with your classification of the codes and themes. Does the reader think that the quotes provided show evidence for the theme in which they are grouped? In this sense, enough quotes should be provided in the analysis section in order for the reader to be able to make this decision. For example, for your 'anxious' theme, you would need to include quotes which adequately explain and show how you came to code these sentences in that way. The reader should be left in no doubt as to why you decided that that sentence revealed the participant to feel anxious about the actions they were about to make. These quotes act as evidence for the conclusions which you have made about how your participants feel.

CONCLUSION

To conclude, qualitative research is a method of collecting and analysing data, it provides the opportunity to meet people and learn first-hand about their experiences and in this way, provides rich, in-depth data. It is also a method, which in a bigger project can be used alongside quantitative methods to add meaning to the results. A final tip is to remember that qualitative research can be very lengthy and time consuming and so it is best to be organised. Qualitative research can be great fun and we hope you enjoy it.

LEARNING OUTCOMES

After reading this chapter you should have a basic understanding of . . .
- What qualitative research is
- The aims of qualitative research
- How to collect qualitative data – interviews and focus groups
- Making sense of your data
- Ensuring rigour in qualitative research.

REFERENCES AND FURTHER READING

Barbour R S 2003 The newfound credibility of qualitative research? Tales of technical essentialism and co-option. Qualitative Health Research 13:1019–1027.

Drummond A 1996 Research methods for therapists. Chapman & Hall, London.

Finlay L, Ballinger C 2006 Qualitative research for allied health professionals: challenging choices. John Wiley, Hoboken NJ.

Flick U 2006 An introduction to qualitative research. SAGE, London.

Krueger R A, Casey M A 2000 Focus Groups: a practical guide for applied research. SAGE, London.

Mays N, Pope C 1995 Qualitative research: rigour and qualitative research. British Medical Journal 311:109–112.

Murray M, Chamberlain K 1998 Qualitative research in health psychology: developments and directions. Journal of Health Psychology 3:291–295.

Richardson J T E 2000 Handbook of qualitative research methods for psychology and the social sciences. The British Psychology Society, Leicester.

Robson C 1997 Real world research: a resource for social scientist and practitioner researchers. Blackwell, Oxford.

Seale J, Barnard S 1998 Therapy research: processes and practicalities. Butterworth Heinemann, London.

Wilkinson S, Joffe H, Yardley L 2004 Qualitative data collection: interviews and focus groups. In: Marks D F, Yardley L (eds) Research methods for clinical and health psychology. SAGE, London.

INDEX